JUICY SEX

By Emma Honey

Contents

Introduction

Everybody needs juicy sex. Even if you and your lover are in perfect harmony, there is scope for creativity – for uncovering secret desires, exploring erotic possibilities, or fulfilling deeply-held wishes. And if you're not happy with your sex life, now is the time to make it better.

Most people want better sex, but often we don't do much about it. There's often a huge rush during the early, passionate stages of the relationship where we explore all sorts of erotic possibilities and (hopefully) find quite a few that work. We all have different sexual styles and varying sexual histories which we bring in to any relationship, and finding out how these are going to work together is an important part of unveiling your sexuality with a new partner.

After a while we often settle into a routine which, although it might be emotionally fulfilling, can become a little humdrum. Sometimes, so-called 'lazy sex' – of the kind where you know what your partner wants, and how to give it to them – is a deliciously intimate and rewarding. The Sunday morning variety, for instance, where you're both making the moves whilst your both still half asleep, and then you're engaged in gentle, dreamy intercourse before you've had time to say 'Good Morning'.

But at other times 'lazy sex' can take on a different meaning, with one partner or the other showing a lack of enthusiasm or even indifference. Under pressure from work, family life or other stresses, your sex life as a couple dwindles. In the long term, passion can wane and frustration sets it, sometimes causing ripples in the relationship – or even ruptures, as one or other partner looks for the expression of their sexual needs elsewhere.

It needn't be this way. The joyous expression of sex is a crucial ingredient in generating intimacy and natural bonding.

But, like anything else that brings a reward, sometimes it takes a little bit of work. I honestly believe that if we invested as much time and energy in sex as we do in shopping or watching television, we'd all be much happier and healthier people. Which is why I've written this book.

"Be adventurous about trying out anything that appeals to you both. Adopt an attitude of playful openness. Through lovemaking you can mutually discover new aspects of yourselves that you had excluded from your sexual identities, bringing you self-acceptance and peace".

Cassandra Lorius *Tantric Secrets*.

Deep and erotic

The purpose of *Juicy Sex* is to break out of the routine and discover the deeper erotic potential in your partnership. It doesn't matter how long you've been together – whether it's 21 days or 21 years – the book is designed to deepen and strengthen your sexual bonding. The core concepts and suggestions can transform your sex life as well as your attitude to each other.

This doesn't mean that you have to drop everything that you were doing previously. In fact, it's important that you don't, because there is some comfort in old patterns and it's okay to be reassured by the familiar – the quickie before you go out for the evening, or the leisurely and languid love-making of a weekend lie-in.

Even if you don't immediately abandon your old habits, one thing which you really must bring to the party is an open mind. You need to be able to stretch your imagination, to take a leap of faith beyond your current mind-set.

We aren't born with sexual skills, they're learned over time. As you try out the techniques and skills in *Juicy Sex* you'll keep some experiences as part of your repertoire, make improvements and adjustments to those you enjoy, and discard others.

The more ideas that you try out, whether individually or 'mixing them up', the richer your sex life will be. The aim is to increase your sex play options, develop new sexual skills, and create higher and longer levels of desire. This in turn will strengthen the intimate, physical bonds between you and your partner so that you can both enjoy a better relationship.

Juicy Sex will open up channels of communication – with yourself, with your partner, and with the erotic universe – which will enrich your being. Life's too short to pass by the chance to experience as many aspects of your sexuality as fully as you can.

Although primarily aimed at heterosexual couples, *Juicy Sex* will be useful for anybody of any sexual orientation. Even if you're not currently with a partner, if you embark on this work – of being in the 'now' of your own sexuality – it will help to change your approach when you <u>are</u> in a loving relationship.

The book is designed to facilitate the conscious exploration of your own and your partner's sexuality. The goal is to tap into that reservoir of sexual power and passion which is already inside you.

I want you to discover that warm, sexy person inside yourself. I'm going to show you how to reach down and grab that sexy beast, and to let loose your erotic instincts - your fabulous sexy self. *Juicy Sex* is about nurturing that inner fire, and unveiling your heaven-sent, glorious sensuality and burning sexual passion.

"You can emerge from shyness into full, lively, rich sexuality - but to get there you'll have to follow your own path, guided by cues from your fantasy life and subconscious".

Carol Queen *Exhibitionism for the Shy*.

What is juicy sex?

It sounds like an obvious question, but it's still worth asking because in so doing, you're asking yourself where your desires lie.

If you're a man, it might be the moment when your heart races as

as your partner turns down the lights and unveils the new lingerie she's bought for herself.

If you're a woman, maybe it's what makes you wet when he touches you with tenderness and passion.

Juicy sex is what makes your scalp prickle as your partner caresses you in exactly the spot you've asked for - whether it's the underside of his balls or the inside of her labia.

It's what makes you want to purr with pleasure when you're on the giving end, and you can feel your partner hum beneath your fingers as if you're playing a well-tuned instrument. It's what makes you moan for more, whether it's being filled up with cock or pleasured with wet pussy.

Sometimes we have hints of our deeper side. There's often a moment where, either through luck or good judgement, something happens differently during sex. Often this is accidental; sometimes it merely comes about through a playful attitude (which is one of the best ways of discovering the depths of your own and your partner's sexuality).

But you need to seize the moment. Sometimes things go so right that we feel we're opening a window into another dimension of our own sexuality, our partner's sexuality, or our joint mingling.

The secret of juicy sex is discovering your sweet spot and then finding a way to bring that fantasy into reality (provided, of course, that it's consensual and doesn't involve harm to other people).

Think about sex scenes from books or films which really get you going, raising your blood pressure and making your heart beat faster. What turns you on? How can you reach that place? Is that passionate explosion between two (or more) people within the realms of the possible for you and your partner?

The people who are making this happen for each other are those who are most deeply linked to their own sexual souls, who have a taproot down to their most personal needs and desires – and it's in this strong mind/body connection that creative sex flourishes.

The goal is to arrive at a space within ourselves that has been called 'the forever place' – the moment where you just want it to go on forever and ever and ever. You want to be in the eternal, blissful 'now' of juicy sex.

"I've learned that sexuality is very fluid and that lines blur (especially in the presence of an experience partner) with little effort. I've come to appreciate the power of sexual arousal and ecstasy to transform people, to heal their spirits, to radically alter their consciousness permanently and for the better. Sexual contact reaches into the depths of a person, transmitting more information in a single moment than can be communicated in any other way"

Nina Hartley *Women Who Ride the Sexual Frontier.*

Know yourself

Knowing yourself is the start of it all. It's not always a straightforward journey to get there: some people make the transition easily, whilst others find that there are emotional or psychological barriers to be overcome. Either way, you have taken the first step by reading this book: the aim is to help you and your partner achieve a state of passion you've never reached before, to be totally fulfilled sexually.

Reaching that point requires letting go of preconceptions, past hurts, and (sometimes) cultural norms. It requires you to open up – not just to yourself, but to your partner as well.

It also requires a degree of emotional vulnerability, of opening up to your feminine side (for men) and masculine side (for women).

Some writers refer to this as our 'sexual intelligence'. The more real, the more vulnerable, and the closer to our real selves that we get, the greater is our sex intelligence.

> "Your sexuality is contained not just in your five physical senses but also in the inner senses of your mind and heart, and the journey to your Inner Goddess begins not with your lover or some esoteric technique but within the private realm of your fantasies, heartfelt desires, daydreams and self-created images about who you are"
>
> Olivia St Claire *227 Ways to Unleash the Sex Goddess in Every Woman.*

Self-knowledge is just the beginning. But what if, in uncovering our own sex intelligence, we were to re-define our erotic selves? Being playful, playing with boundaries, playing with new erotic ideas: these are key concepts for tuning into your own sex intelligence. What *is* really kinky? Who's to say?

Why not inject some fantasy, erotic literature, or role-playing into your love life? Playing around with new skills or ideas will help you develop your sex intelligence alongside your bedroom repertoire. This is what keeps it fresh and keeps it passionate. It's the beginning of a dialogue which will last you a lifetime.

And remember that there's no one 'correct' way to be in your own sexuality; both you and your partner will have changing needs which will evolve over time in response to different stimuli – the state of your relationship, the ageing process, the time or day/month/year and so forth.

Good sex is about what's wanted by either or both partners at a particular moment: its being aware of those needs which makes for the juiciest sex and developing the most intimate bonds.

It goes without saying that you should always practice safe sex, and that everything you do must be consensual (that is, both partners agree to it). Apart from that, it's up to you—enjoy!

Chapter One: Let's Talk Sex

Good communication is the key to juicy, creative sex. Sharing your thoughts on what you want, your likes and dislikes (plus of course where you draw the line in bedroom antics) will vastly improve your sex life.

It seems curious to me that some couples are content to spend hours on end discussing important topics which will affect the quality of their lives – decorating the house, say, or where to go on holiday – but don't talk much about sex. This is gradually changing over time, but there's still an element of taboo about expressing our sexual selves to each other, and being able to talk about it.

It's as if we expect communication around sex to take place by some kind of magical wish fulfillment, without any conscious effort on our part.

All good relationships are founded on good communication, and that includes being open and honest around sex. The sooner you start this conversation, the better. During the early stages of a relationship you're probably bonking like rabbits and everything's fine, but sooner or later you'll need to start learning about each other's sexuality in more depth. If you leave it too long it's likely to be too late because the long you take, the more awkward it becomes.

Trust your partner and express yourself. Be upfront, it usually works. Even just slipping in the odd hint when you first get to know each other can help create the impression of you as an open, liberated lover.

Your own needs and wants will also change over time, and it'll be easier to discuss this if you've been talking openly from the beginning.

There are many reasons why people don't start this conversation. It could be from shyness, or not wanting to seem slutty (women), or being stuck with the strong, silent label (men). A major factor is anxieties around not wanting to hurt each other's feelings.

If you've never discussed sex with your partner then break the ice by mentioning the fact that you find it difficult to discuss sex (whether you do or don't), but it matters to you and you'd like to take the first step towards more open communication.

As your partner becomes aware that it's okay to discuss these kinds of issues, your knowledge of each other – and your sex intelligence within the relationship- will continue to grow. As you get to know each other better and you reveal your likes and dislikes, you'll build greater trust and be rewarded with a relationship where you feel safe to explore the deeper layers of your sexual soul.

It really is important to start as you mean to go on: if you can get the dialogue going early on, your partner will have a picture of you as liberated and fun – and will be more open to accept your suggestions. But if you act totally straight-laced in the bedroom from

Day One, it can be tricky to get the conversation going further down the line.

It may also be helpful in identifying basic incompatibilities: sometimes we find that, however hard we try, our partner's sexual style just doesn't match our own. Sometimes you can find a way around this – but sometimes not.

Lovers who identify incompatibilities in this way will need to try and discover what they do share and find some other way to satisfy the desires they don't share.

It's far simpler to discover what erotic activities are most important to you, and find a partner who shares those needs, early on in the relationship. Revealing deeply-held sexual secrets to a long-term partner can have its own complications.

By keeping or special needs, fantasies and fetishes a secret, we're only hurting ourselves. Being open and honest means that we not only enjoy more pleasure, but we're able to revel in exactly that type of pleasure which is unique to us – our own sexual signature, the essence of our deeper sexual selves. This is what reaching for juicier sex is all about.

Be positive

Being positive and encouraging your lover to keep doing whatever it is that you're enjoying is one of the best ways to educate your partner about what you do like (as opposed to what you don't like). 'Yes' is such a good word in these circumstances – it can have so many intonations, so many different ways of being emphasized.

> "The best sex is between two people who come to the bedroom fully informed about their own needs and desires. They know what gets them off and how they liked to be touched and where. You're not going to get very far if either of you thinks the other should know just what they want. So it's up to you to make sure you do know what you like, and then communicate those desires to your lover. The more you are in touch with what gets you hot, the better you will be able to show your lover how to please you".

Candida Royale *How to Tell A Naked Man What Do.*

'Yes yes yes!'

Most people want to give their partners as much pleasures as possible, and if we can learn to express our needs without judgement or anger it's much easier to get what we want. If we leave it too long, changing your sexual persona further down the line can be much more difficult. So start as you mean to go on – once you begin to open up, both of you will become more liberated and accepting of each other's sexual preferences.

Encouragement rather than criticism is important. The key is to say things in a way which makes your partner feel loved and appreciated. Be positive – for instance, "I love the way you touch me, but could you

do it a little higher/lighter/harder/softer..please?".
Make sure you acknowledge their response, as in "Oh
yes, just like that", or "That feels incredible".

Warm, breathy words will go a lot further than a cold,
hard 'Don't do that!".

Moaning, groaning, or your own reciprocal touch are
other ways of giving feedback. Warm, breathy words
are good. Let them know when they hit a sweet spot.
"Don't stop, that's perfect, keep doing that", are all
good expressions.

As each of you reveals a layer, one after the other, you
will build greater trust and develop a relationship
where you can explore the deepest and richest thrills
of eroticism as well as the lighter, playful side of sex.

Slow hand, light touch.

Getting down to specifics can also be helpful. "I'm
going to try this, and then that - tell me which you like
best" is one way of discovering your lover's
preferences.

A gentle hint to move a hand, to suggest a lighter or
heavier touch, or to ask for a position you want can
move the action instantly on to a more highly-charged
erotic plane.

Learning how to do this in a way that makes your
partner feel valued and cherished is an essential part
of being a creative lover. Ask your partner to talk you
through their responses: make it a game, ask them to
kiss you in a way they would like to be kissed, or to

run your hands over their body how they would like it done.

Groan and moan to get the message across. Vocalisation is hugely important. Responding with 'Yes, yes!' to the right touch, or 'Please don't stop that', will encourage your partner but contribute to your own arousal.

Sometimes one word is better 'softer', 'harder', 'up', or 'down'. Loosening up your vocal chords, moaning, groaning and talking during sex, is a great way of releasing sexual energy.

Use open-ended questions, such as: "What would you like me to do which would really turn you on?", or "How can I give you more pleasure?"

Don't assume your lover is a mind reader, clued up on your wants and desires. I think women in particular are guilty of assuming men are going to be tuned into their body and to automatically know what they need in bed; this goes hand-in-hand with the assumption that orgasms (his and hers) are the man's responsibility. It places an unfair burden on the poor guy to keep both of you sexually fulfilled and can lead to resentment if this doesn't happen. Women need to play an equal part by making their preferences known, and finding out what pleases their lover.

"We all have little sex sounds we use during love-making and you can use these to better affect for communication. Those sighs, moans and groans are important signals to let you lover know how much you're enjoying something. The more you want them to do something the more noise you should make. It's also important to listen carefully to their sex-sounds. Listen and learn, and apply this to what you are doing to them".

Pam Spurr *Sensational Sex*.

The 'yes' session

Try this as a pick-me-up if you feel your sex life is stuck in a rut, or as a way of finding out more about what your partner likes and doesn't like. Agree in advance that you'll try and get each other to say 'yes' as many times as possible during love-making (although you're not planning to count them – this isn't a competition!). Use it as an opportunity to explore new ways of touching each other, with no embarrassment if it goes wrong or your partner doesn't like what you're doing. Just simply say 'yes', with varying degrees of emphasis, in response to things your partner is doing which you do like. You'll find there are dozens of different ways of saying 'yes' (and some hurdles, of course, if you're both using your mouths on each other). With any luck you may end up simultaneously screaming 'Yes! Yes! Yes!' together in climax.

The ecstasy rating system

A good way to communicate with each other is with an 'ecstasy rating' system, which is basically grading anything that you're doing to each other on a scale of one to ten In response to a 'Do you like that?' query. The answer might be a four: it's nice but not sending me up the wall; six or seven might be hitting nearer the spot; or a nine would be approaching orgasmic. Once you initiate this, you'll find it's a great feedback system for any sexual activity you try. You'll find yourselves escalating up the number scale together—a terrific erotic feedback loop.

Share a 'wish list'

Make your wants known – drop hints, start to open the door. Keep your antennae tuned to your partner's needs, and learn to listen out for clues. Make suggestions – perhaps you're watching a sexy film, or you've read something kinky in a book – then let your partner know you'd like to try it out.

Visiting a sex shop together is another great way to be able to share and explore together. Many of these are now specifically female- or couple-friendly in a way that old-style sex shops usually weren't.

Browsing on-line sex stores, kinky clothing outlets, or other websites can also help communications (some, such as LoveHoney.com, operate a wish list which you can share with your partner. This is a fantastic way of flagging up things that you'd like to explore together).

So make your wishes known, whether it's by email, text, or a whispered confession in the ear: and if you're the recipient, treasure these requests coming from your lover's deepest heart. Savour them, play with them, and build on them: prepare to create a truly explosive experience for you both. One of the most flattering things you can do for a person is to adjust your repertoire when you've learned what their sexual preferences are.

Be open-minded

As you and your partner start to be more adventurous and open up to each other, it may throw up a few surprises. Try and keep an open mind, and not be too judgemental. A sense of humour is important - laughing with someone is fine, but laughing at them is just cruel. If you're presented with a request or scenario that you've never thought of before, at least give your partner credit for trying to spice things up a bit. If it's really outside your comfort zone, you need to be able to discuss it and reach a compromise about what you will or won't do.

Most sex play is intrinsically benign, as long as it doesn't involve pain of any kind (unless it's deliberate pain, as in BDSM). If something your partner has suggested is really not for you, then you need to make that clear at the outset – and find out whether they can live without it or not.

This is another reason why you should talk sex early on: if someone's sexual style isn't going to suit you, then its best that you both discover this incompatibility at an early stage. Those with very kinky or fetishistic behaviours now find it much easier to find compatible partners through the internet, so if that's important to you, you're better off looking somewhere else. If you know what erotic activities make you happy, it's easier to find someone to share them with.

Open, courageous communication is essential for juicy sex. Once this process begins, you're creating the conditions for a lifetime of dialogue and sexual empowerment.

Safe sex

It's important that you discuss safe sex before you begin to have sex with a new partner. Difficult though it may be, it will make for a much more relaxed and enjoyable encounter. If you feel you can't broach the subject, reconsider having sex with that person.

Getting more of what you want

"We keep our fantasies, our fetishes, and our special needs a secret. If we were more open and honest we'd not only enjoy more pleasure, we'd enjoy the type of pleasure which is special and unique to us. We don't say that we don't like a certain touch and we rarely say what type of touch we do like. We kiss, but without detailing the intricacies of kissing which are especially delicious.

We ignore our own discomfort or displeasure because we fear insulting or hurting our partner. We neglect to say what we want, how we want it. And when we want it. We allow a special moment to pass rather than intrude on feelings or ego. We actually deprive ourselves in deference to our beliefs that we have to protect our lovers from the humiliations of requests or corrections.

Most of the time our beliefs are unfounded. If we learn how to express ourselves without judgement or anger, we can actually get what we want without unpleasant repercussions".

Carol Altman *Sex Talk*

Chapter Two: Setting the Scene

Juicy Bedrooms

Juicy sex can take place anywhere but for most of us, most of the time, sex takes place in the bedroom. So what does yours look like? Are you surrounded by piles of ironing, redundant exercise machines, discarded books and an abandoned cat basket? Is it a sexy space? Probably not.

It's time to create a juicier atmosphere. Maybe you're in the first throes of passionate love and don't care where you make love but, for the rest of us, sex is better in a boudoir-like setting. Boring surroundings make for boring sex, while a sensuous environment sets the stage for heightened sexual experiences.

So it's well worth investing time and effort into turning your bedroom into a place of hot sensuality, a suitable backdrop for your amorous adventures. All it takes is a little effort and imagination. You don't need to spend a lot of money: tap into your own creativity if you're short of cash.

If you're not yet in a relationship, then start by creating the sort of room where you expect it all to happen. Make the space right, and it *will* happen.

The Karma Sutra advises that your room should be "balmy with rich perfumes, and contain a soft bed, agreeable to the sight, covered with a clean, white cloth, having garlands and bunches of flowers upon it, and two pillows, one at the top and one at the bottom".

You might not be able to re-create this ideal of an oriental seraglio but you can make a start by de-cluttering: get an extra wardrobe if necessary, and get clothes out of sight. Get rid of cuddly toys, laundry baskets, crappy old posters, piles of shoes, etc etc. Some form of music is good, all other electronics (particularly laptops – unless you're watching something hot!) should be banished.

Think about how you're going to combine colours and textures to create a warmer, softer atmosphere. Give the walls a coat of paint – go for single, deep colours such as plum or burgundy. Re-cover cushions or duvets in touchy-feely fabrics such as velvet, suede, sheepskin, satin, fake fur or chenille (scour second-hand shops for old velvet curtains, or see what you can find on Ebay). Splash out on some deep, richly-coloured curtains or rugs.

"Sometimes [fulfilling your fantasies] is as easy as a purchase. What material will do this for you? What scent? What colour? What sound? Make it happen. Buy it and use it: allow it, whatever it is, to augment and intensify your sexual pleasures. Free your mind and your thoughts, allow them to soar, to explode, and to become your reality. Your sexual reality will roar with the addition of dreamed moments and fantasized sensations".

Carole Altman *Sex Talk*.

Re-calibrate your lighting to give a softer look; light switches should be easily controllable from the bed. Make niches for plenty of candles (preferably safely placed in glass holders – particularly those next to the bed, which might take a spill when the action gets passionate). Make a special place for an oil-burner for essential essences, or incense sticks.

A bedroom TV is an acceptable way to lure someone under the covers, so make sure it's visible from the bed and the remote control is handy.

If you can manage it, create a canopy over the bed (search on-line for 'bed canopy': there are plenty of low-priced options). This creates a very intimate, private space within the bedroom: a sort of room-within-a-room.

Even better is a four-poster bed, which has the same effect: very private and cosy, enclosing you and your partner in your own little juicy shared nirvana.

The toy box

"At the head of the couch should be a sort of stool, on which should be placed the fragrant ointments for the night", says the Karma Sutra. Yes, this means that lubes, condoms and other accessories should be easily available so it's useful to have a handy drawer or bedside cabinet to keep lubricants, condoms, and basic sex toys within close reach. In a shared or family home, it's also sensible if this is lockable. As your repertoire expands and your inventory of sex toys increases, you might want to create an adult toy box. You can easily adapt this from something bought second-hand, like an old trunk (paint it to match your new décor). Again, keep your whips, handcuffs and fantasy uniforms under lock and key if necessary.

Create a love nest

Whilst you're giving the bedroom a make-over, consider investing in a new set of bed linen. Your bedroom should be an invitation to naked sensuality – and that includes the bed sets. Soft cotton sheets are always good (the higher the thread count, the better – although these are more expensive). However, splurging on something a little more exotic will make a definitive statement about your erotic intentions (yes! Juicy sex here we come!).

- Silk is of course massively sensual and luxurious, although comparatively expensive.

Try on-line retailers such as jasminesilk.com or duvetandpillowwarehouse.co.uk

- Satin is a completely acceptable alternative, and much cheaper. There are some extremely good value satin bed sets available on-line at sites such as linensdirect.co.uk

- Bamboo bed linen is a new trend – the fabric wicks away moisture, so it's cool in summer and warm in winter. It's also incredibly soft and silky, and sustainably grown to boot. betweenthesheets.co.uk has the first 100% bamboo bedding range in the UK (including duvet covers, sheets, pillowcases, valences) available in all bed sizes. Their bamboo used a special weave for softness and durability and although it only has a 250 thread count it feels softer than 1000 thread-count cotton.

Now for some of the kinkier stuff – and this is really signalling an intention to invest in your sex life and delve deeper in your fantasies.

- The ultimate in fetish fantasy is the latex bed sheet. These rubber sheets usually come in red or black and yes they are expensive, with a standard fitted double sheet priced at £150 plus: for the whole set (sheet, duvet cover and couple of pillow cases) you're looking at over £400. But if properly maintained they'll last a long time – and you can have an awful lot of fun even with just one double sheet. The *look* and the *feel* are all about sensuality: slipping and sliding with your lubricated partner, skin-on-rubber, skin-on-skin, rubber-on-skin: that's an erotic experience I think is well worth the money (make sure your lubes and oils are water-based, though). It's not something we do everyday, and to be honest you can't really sleep on latex (it gets hot and sweaty). Check betweenthesheets.co.uk

- Another option is high-gloss polyurethane coated sheets ('high gloss PU'). This is another sensational tactile experience, and (unlike latex) this fantastic bedding won't be damaged by non-aqueous massage oils and lubricants. PU High Gloss is actually polyurethane (which gives the high gloss finish) on strong, stretchy polyester jersey. They're ideal for fun play and come in a much wider range of colours than latex. They're also sensational for Nuru Gel massage (see page 138).

Dressing for Sex

Lingerie can be a potent part of juicy sex. Wearing sensuous underwear can be a real catalyst in creating desire in both you and your partner.

Silks and satins, for instance, hold a tantalising allure for both men and women. There's something about the smooth, lustrous sheen that makes you want to caress the fabric and, naturally enough, the person wearing it. Made from finely-woven silk, satin and satin-type materials feel sexy next to bare skin and can be an inexpensive alternative to silk.

Shop or browse catalogues or internet sites together, choosing items which will turn you both on. Pandering to each others' preferences shows that you're attentive to your partners' sexual needs, will help you understand the desires of your partner and will fuel your libidos.

Half the fun of lingerie lies in not taking it off altogether. The partial revelation—the glimpse of breast or thigh revealed—can be just as arousing, and the sense of touch—silk, softness, satin, and skin—is heightened if they continue through sex.

"Underwear clings to our most private parts...underthings taunt, tease, stroke and caress. Our underwear goes places that no other item can reach, curving, bending, and moistening as we do. Our underwear is a barometer for our lust, enhancing our pleasure by teasing us with its presence. Stroking a hard dick or a wet pussy through someone's underwear is a tease – you're so near and yet so far. Sometimes almost-nude is hotter than totally naked".

Rachel Kramer Bussel *Ultimate Undies: Erotic Stories About Underwear and Lingerie.*

Don't just take your partners underwear off, push the material aside with your tongue, tug it with your teeth, tease around the seams. Drape panties around male genitalia during sex, tease nipples through a sexy bra or bustier, or finger your lover's sex through satin panties. Again, don't be afraid to experiment until you find what you both like.

Incorporate sexy underwear into your role-playing fantasies, or for hot date nights, whether for sexy dancing, stripping, or just lolling around by the fireside enjoying a sensual, sexy cuddle.

"Lingerie is transformative, as are clothes. Allow yourself the freedom to let go and become the vixen you want to be. Be creative and play. The bedroom is the one place we get to be both playful and grown up. Got with it and most of all, have fun!"

Candida Royale *How to Tell a Naked Man What to Do*.

For her:

Take your partner to a quality lingerie shop or specialist ladies erotica store and insist that he choose at least one item that he'd like to see you wearing. Most men don't need much persuasion to help their partner choose lingerie!

If you buy more than one item, try to be varied to keep interest aroused. Stockings are classic and affordable and always please. In fact, anything that covers but gives a (big) hint of flesh is ideal, such as corsets and bustiers (though these can be more expensive).

In the underwear department, less is more—skimpy, frivolous, wispy, and frilly bits all hold the promise of hidden delights for your lover. Black is classically wicked and sophisticated, white signals virginal innocence, and red is for outright naughtiness. Remember that attraction, for males, is visual so make an effort and show yourself off.

As a surprise, treat yourself and your partner to some shamelessly expensive lingerie from retailers such as AgentProvocateur.com, or myla.com. It might leave you out of pocket but he'll thank you until his tongue aches.

> "Think of yourself as a present. It's what's inside that truly counts but the presentation can have him eagerly tearing back those layers to get to what lies beneath. When you look fantastic, you feel fantastic, which will have you exuding confidence and sex appeal in spades"
>
> Lexie Sutton *Fifty Shades of Bliss*

For him:

Men's underwear can and should be just as erotic as women's: every man should have a good selection of sexy underwear designed for play time in the bedroom.

Men like to feel desirable, attractive, sexy and sophisticated just as much as women do, and the range of really sexy underwear made for men is increasing all the time - led by designers at BodyAware.com and Planet-Undies.com, amongst others. Gay stores such as Clone Zone (clonezonedirect.com) have a much sexier range of jockstraps and underwear than anything you'll find in Ann Summers. You'll also find an excellent selection of strings, thongs and top male underwear brands such as Hom available on-line at deadgoodundies.com

What could be more alluring than a man who has dressed with seduction (and undressing) on his mind?

There's more to choose from than you might think. If you're new to this, you'll be amazed at some of the different styles available, from stripper thongs to J-strings, slingshots, straps, and much more.

Get ready to express yourself in silk, satin, latex, leather, pvc, and many other sexy fabrics. Try out some thongs, G-strings, shorts or jockstraps with your partner or play on your own. Get lots of attention by showing off your muscular assets beneath a net vest. Why should women have all the fun?

Silks and satins feel just as gorgeous wrapped around his genitals as they do around hers. Get your lover to help you choose several items with sex appeal, or surprise her next time she unzips your jeans.

Give yourselves permission to play: stroking through silk, tugging at a thong, playing with pouches adds another element to sex, whether on your own or with a partner. It increases stimulation around the perineum, anus and your balls (especially in conjunction with a cock ring).

Make sure that you feel comfortable or else you won't feel sexy. For this reason avoid cheap, scratchy fabrics (exactly the same rule applies to women's lingerie) and whatever you do, stay away from 'joke' jock straps with animal faces on them. The Ann Summers chain is particularly bad at catering for adult tastes in this respect.

Juicy Scent

The reason that Inuit peoples rub noses instead of kissing is because they find the scent of their lovers' breath more erotic than the taste of their saliva. Consciously you might be aware of your partner's perfume or cologne but subconsciously your brain will be analysing their personal odour.

Smell is the quickest route to the brain—it takes just two seconds from nose to sensory receptors to the limbic centres that control emotions. A man's hot, well-exercised body exuding clean, fresh sweat is a real turn-on for some women. Equally, the female body's unwashed odour (*la cassolette*, in French, meaning 'perfume box'), which comes from hair, body odours, armpits, and genitals, is just as attractive to men.

Everyone's body has its own unique scent: a hormonal mix that is carried by pheromones from yourself to those around you. These 'information carriers' let other people know your sexual state. Subconsciously your mind will analyse this information very rapidly, leading to a decision as to whether or not you are attracted to them. If you have a sensitive nose you can often detect pheromones whilst kissing your lover.

For her: According to Ayurvedic principles the female sex drive is governed by the lower abdomen. Dabbing fragrances on the stomach then as foreplay increases the blood flow and generates heat to release their erotic aromas. Some people claim that lavender oil behind the ears is a guaranteed man-puller, although others swear that vaginal juices judiciously applied to a woman's neck or torso will attract men, even though the men won't know what they're reacting to.

For him: Good grooming is essential. Take good care of your appearance and make sure that you smell attractive. Try various colognes, body sprays, body oils and creams (but not all at the same time!). Those blended specially to encourage intimacy come from elements of lavender and oak moss which give off woody, musky base notes which are said to generate intimacy.

Lubricants

Good sex is slippery and awash with body fluids including saliva, sweat and secretions. Lubricants create temporary, extra wetness and come in all shapes and sizes, from a tube of jelly to a small sachet of fruity liquid. You can buy basic lubricant from the chemist or visit a sex store for greater variety.

When to use lube

Hormones, alcohol, and stress can prevent natural lubrication and this is where lube comes in useful, to give nature a hand. Lubricant can be a pleasant accessory to masturbation for both men and women.

Vibrators and dildos almost always require lubrication. For either sex, lubrication is an absolute must for anal play—even just inserting a finger—because the rectum does not self-lubricate and dry insertions can cause damage.

Choosing lube

Any sex shop, erotica catalogue or on-line store will feature a wide range of lubricants. But how do you decide which one is best for you? Oil-based lubes (ranging from coconut to mineral or vegetable oils) have been in use for centuries but they can create irritation, or allergic reactions in the body. They can also damage any latex products that you are using, from condoms and diaphragms, to dildos and vibrators. In the case of the former, rendering them ineffective. Avoid these.

Water-based lubricants are generally the safest all-round lubricants. They won't harm latex and will wash out of you (and your sheets) with ease. Water-based lubes tend to lose their slippery quality relatively quickly but you can easily reactivate them by adding water (keep a glass by the bed).

Silicone lubricants are formulated to be more slippery and to last longer before drying out and becoming too sticky. Although they are also water-based and safe to use with latex, they can damage silicone sex toys. You can partially avoid this by using a condom on your silicone toys. Silicone lubes are more expensive than purely water-based ones with the price usually reflecting concentration.

Choosing lubricant depends upon the type you enjoy using and what you're using it for. The drier the area where the lubricant is being used, the thicker the lubricant should be, for example, use thin liquid lube to stimulate the clitoris where there are already some natural juices, a thicker lubricant for dildos. Some lubricants demonstrate 'sheer thinning', that is, the faster you move, the more slippery it becomes. A good sex shop or on-line store should be able to give you the information on type and suitability so don't be afraid to ask. Because most lubricants contain chemicals, even many flavoured lubes are unpleasant to have in your mouth. Again, ask for advice in the shop or check out brands on-line that are suitable for licking.

Some lubricants contain the contraceptive agent, nonoxynol-9, intended to increase the efficiency of condoms as contraceptives. Be aware that this agent can cause an allergic reaction on the skin. Similarly, glycerine, common in water-based lubes, can also upset sensitive skin.

Natural lubes

If you'd prefer to avoid unnatural ingredients altogether then try lubes from a company called Yes. Their lubes have no synthetic chemicals in them, they're based on totally natural ingredients, and they're also good for your skin. yesyesyes.org

Your sex toy box:

Check out any decent on-line sex store and you soon realise that the variety and range of sex toys available in the market today is amazing, and the choices incredible. Try lovehoney.co.uk, annsummers.com or sh-womenstore.com

Vibrators & Dildos

The dildo was original sex toy, used by the Baylonians, Greeks and Romans, centuries ago. A dildo is any penis-shaped object, designed for vaginal or anal insertion. In ancient times they were made from ivory, stone or wood but are now made from rubber, silicone or latex and are available in a huge range of colours, textures and sizes.

Probably the first new sex toy to be invented after the dildo, vibrators are one of the most popular bedroom accessories with dozens of different styles available. The simplest are battery-operated, often explicitly penis-shaped. They're cheaper to buy than electric ones but are generally less powerful than their electric counterparts. Vibrators come in huge range of sizes and colours, from the classic Rabbit to tiny, lipstick-shaped ones which you can hide in a handbag for those unexpected surprises during a night out.

There are plenty of ways to be creative with vibrators, whether you're using them for masturbating yourself or your partner or using them in sex play. They feel good used as a massage tool, and they're useful for discovering hidden erogenous zones. Hands-free vibrators come in various shapes and sizes, including the 'butterfly' type that can be strapped on, either for use during intercourse or solo sex.

Don't feel you need to have only one, or only one type. If you have two, you can use them on each other simultaneously, or use a vibrator inside a lover's vagina and use another on her clit. There are egg-shaped vibrators, designed to be inserted vaginally but they can also be used to stimulate the clitoris. Some vibrators are specially shaped in order to reach the female G Spot whilst others are curved to maximise massage on the male prostrate. Handiest of all are the small 'clit-buzzers' or 'finger-tinglers' that slip on the end of a digit.

"One night when we were out for a special celebration I asked my girlfriend to wear a short skirt and a long coat: after dinner, we went to a very noisy, crowded bar where we kissed and cuddled standing up in a corner. Nothing unusual about that for a Friday night: however, I'd slipped a 'finger tingler' onto my hand and, hidden by her long coat, reached between her legs as we were kissing and chatting. Pretty soon she was gripping my shoulders and staring at me with a wild look in her eyes as I massaged her clit through her knickers with the mini-vibrator. It was so busy and noisy no-one else saw (or heard) a thing! We've never forgotten that evening".

Peter, Bath, 43.

Jiggle Balls: These consist of two small balls, usually linked together, which are inserted into the vagina. They come in a variety of sizes and materials – some are solid, some contain a small weight. The idea is that they roll around together as you move, increasing sensation in the pelvic area. They can also be used to increase the strength of your pelvic floor muscles, like Kegel exercises. Some women find them enjoyable, others find that they do nothing at all for them – how you react may depend on the size of the balls and what you do while you're wearing them

Boys' Toys

There are a huge variety of sex toys available for guys using them on their own or with a partner – however, easily the best selling sex toy for men is the cock ring. Your toy box should be stocked with several different kinds which you can choose according to your mood.

A cock ring is essentially a strap which is worn at the base of the penis and is designed to stop the blood flowing back out once you've got an erection. Theoretically, it will give you a longer and harder erection and it's true that a cock ring will create a harder, more sensitive and more intensive erection – but this doesn't necessarily mean it will last longer. The increased sensation might actually make you come sooner. They will undoubtedly make you feel bigger and harder, and give you a more intense orgasm. A cock ring is also useful if you've already come once, and your next erection needs a bit of help.

There are lots of different types: usually simplest is best, but everyone has different tastes. A proper cock ring goes round the base of your cock and balls. Some are sold to go around the shaft of your penis, but they don't stay on very well or perform quite the same function.

Worn at the base of the scrotum, a cock ring holds your balls away from your body and allowing much more freedom in terms of touching and manipulation.

They stop your testicles migrating back into their body cavities, for a start, so you (or your partner) can play with them much more with less anxiety of being hurt.

- Cock rings with fasteners are generally the easiest to use: either they have snap closings, or Velcro; you can usually pull the snap fasteners nice and tight.

- Vibrating and novelty rings: there's loads of choice here. Usually there's a vibrating bullet which stimulates your testicles or alternatively it's placed to stimulate your partner's clit during sex.

- Gay sex stores have the best selections. Try clonezonedirect.co.uk for everything from classics such as a plain leather cock strap through to more advanced models such as weighted straps, cock cages, ball-stretchers and the like. In the US babeland.com has a useful range from simple Velcro leather straps through to stretchy rubber cock rings.

Sex toy hygiene

It's important that vibrators and dildos should be kept clean and germ free. They should be cleaned with a damp cloth or washed in warm, soapy water. Make sure vibrators and dildos are completely dry before putting them away, to avoid bacterial growth. Never ever use a vibrator or dildo anally and then insert it in the vagina, or vice versa, without cleaning it thoroughly first, because this can create cross-infection. You can use condoms to keep dildos and vibrators hygienic at all times.

Chapter Three: Creative sex play

Invest in yourselves

We tend to spend less time and effort on our sex lives than we do on almost any other areas of our lives: think how much money you spend on food or clothes each week, or how much time you spend on household chores, cooking, watching television or other entertainment. Then think about how much time and energy you invest in your sex life.

Comparatively, it's not very much – about an hour a week, according to surveys. Of course there are innumerable pressures (including work, housework, family commitments and so on) which mean that sex becomes a low priority. But at the same time it seems strange to relegate sex to the bottom of the list of things that you want to do together – especially since the rewards can be so high. Often it becomes just a late night thing, and by then most of us are too tired to care.

And yet - investing in your sex life is as important as getting enough exercise, following a healthy diet, or nurturing your own well being in other ways. Physically, sex is good for you in many different ways, including promoting cardiovascular fitness, increasing oxygen flow to your tissues and organs, lowering cholesterol, and boosting your immune system.

Sex also boosts your mental health by releasing endorphins into the bloodstream, which helps reduce stress and increase feelings of well-being and relaxation. Regular sex can also help boost your oxytocin levels, which also contribute to your emotional health.

If you want to rev up your sex life, I suggest that you agree with your partner to:

1) Set aside the time for regular sex dates, which will give you space to explore juicier sex together.

2) Set a sex budget, which will give you freedom to explore more options for juicier sex together.

The first of these is essential; the second is optional – but desirable. Investing in your sex life – whether creating time, or bringing in other resources - is investing in yourselves.

Make a sex date

The first rule of juicy sex is to make time in your schedules for a sex date. This is one of the most affirmative, positive actions you can take to move your sex life onto another level with each other. Simply the fact of having committed the time and energy to consciously and intentionally explore your sexuality will change your relationship for the better.

Although initially it may seem counter-intuitive (or just plain wrong) that pre-planned sex will be sexy, couples who've practised it for years will tell you it's one of the most important ingredients in creating a lasting, loving bond between them.

Even if regular sex becomes lazy sex, or vanilla sex, or just plain 'I need an orgasm in order to go to sleep' sex, or middle-of-the-week sex, at least you know that something more exciting is on the horizon.

By planning a sex date together you're actively creating the time and space to explore your erotic potential, to spice things up in the bedroom.

Whether you make your date via your smart phone's synchronized calendar, write a perfumed note naming the time and place, or simply yell across the kitchen – "Thursday 6pm, OK?!" - the effect is going to be the same. You're building anticipation, wallowing in expectation, thinking juicy thoughts and getting ready for massively hot sex.

It's a shared commitment to erotic satisfaction, and the fact that its set in advance gives it big impetus as an *intention* to have a lot of fun. It doesn't matter whether it's once a week or once a month, the key is in having a regular commitment to erotica time.

"There are many bridges to desire but the most over-looked must be planning. Maybe it is a legacy of our Victorian past but many people are only happy when they are swept away by their emotions – and therefore do not have to take responsibility for their desires. Of course, spontaneous lovemaking is wonderful and exciting, but if you wait until both of you just happen to be in the right mood, at the same time and in the right place…you can end up waiting a long, long time. Alternatively, a little planning can solve all these problems".

Andrew G Marshall *How to Make Love Like a Prairie Vole*.

"My partner treated me to a really sexy, sensual sex date recently. I arrived at his house after a long journey to find a note at the bottom of the stairs telling me not to talk, and to follow the rose petals. The rose petals led me to the bedroom where another note told me to undress, put on an eye mask, and get in the bathtub (which he'd already filled with hot, foamy water). I have a lot of trust in Jeff, which allowed me to surrender to the excitement and suspense of what was to come. He came into the bathroom very quietly, and began to stroke my entire body with a waterproof, vibrating massage glove which he'd bought. It was amazingly smooth and seductive. Then he fed my juicy fruits – strawberries and mangoes – with his fingers and also his mouth. He placed lots of kisses all over my body in the bath. All of this without a word being exchanged between us. There was something very luscious in having my whole body caressed, which led to me enjoying several lovely orgasms. It was one of the most erotic and sensual experiences I have had, and it warms my heart that he put so much effort into creating this experience for me".

Felicity, 28, Leeds.

Be adventurous

As part of your sex dates, commit yourself to trying something new on a regular basis. Whether it's once a week, once a fortnight, or once a month, it doesn't matter. The point of this is to have fun with sex play that you haven't tried before.

It might be an idea from a video, a magazine, a book, or internet site, a new sex toy, or as simply a new item of sexy underwear.

Be adventurous and surprise your partner with something mischievous. If you don't take the risk you might miss out on oceans of delicious pleasure together. Be bold – share your on-line wish list.

Don't be limited by past sexual patterns. Most of us follow an imprint of experiences that were developed during the sexual awakening of our teens. If we don't change this 'erotic map' then we're likely to limit ourselves to a constant repetition of arousal and climax that should have been left behind years ago. Chuck out all your old habits.

Explore new ideas, learn new skills, play games, dress up, read the erotic classics (to yourself, for ideas, and out loud), and enjoy. Remember though; always be gentle with your partner at first until you're sure of your touch and their preferences.

Sometimes experimenting with new ideas, toys, clothes, roles, fantasies or anything else involved in juicy sex play can feel strange. Don't give up if a new technique doesn't work first time. Try it at least three times—twice while you figure out precisely how things should be, and on the third time it should all click into place. If either you or your partner feel uncomfortable, and it's not just first-time nerves, then just move on to a new idea. You must remember, however, that there are some things that you might try which are just not for you.

Here's a good exercise for you and your partner that will allow you both to start to explore your boundaries. Each of you should grab pen and paper and write down your answers to the following:

- All the things you would like to try.

- All the things you definitely don't want to do.

- Everything in between, such as areas you're not sure of but *might* like to explore.

Sit down with your partner, swap papers and discuss and, with the minimum of embarrassment, start to get an idea of each other's more hidden desires. An alternative to this is to write a list of five things you'd like your lover to do to you and, once again, swap lists.

Try and project yourself into your lover's head (or their loins...). What scent will turn him on? What colour does she love? What material would feel good for both of us? Go for it - pluck that fantasy out of the ether and make it happen, turning sexual dreams into erotic reality.

Another route into this is through the kind of games (available on-line) such as Nookie, Kama Sutra cards, or 'love dice' which direct you to do different things to your lover on the role of a dice.

Uninterrupted time (kids away, mobiles turned off) is also important.

Set a Sex Budget

Create a sex budget by deciding with your partner that you're going to spend x amount per week, or per month, on things to spice up your sex lives. You can budget for anything from sex toys to self-indulgent weekends away. Or you could decide to turn your bedroom into a sexy nook.

The more you invest in your sex life, the more you'll get out of it. By introducing new things into the bedroom, whether its lingerie, erotic books, or sex toys, you're creating new kinetic and sensual experiences to share with each other, and opening up new avenues of communication between you.

The process of deciding what techniques, ideas, sex toys or other sensual pleasures to introduce into the bedroom (or kitchen, bathroom….) will in itself help you develop a more adventurous attitude.

Keep your sexual antennae alert to your partner's desires. Is there a hint in something they're telling you? Is there some chance comment which you could delve further into?

You'll be amazed at some of the things which excite people, but try not to be judgmental—it might be your partner who's getting goose bumps imagining what *that* is used for. Keep an open mind, and keep your sexual antennae tuned. Make a game of it where each of you has to choose at least one item that you think the other would like to wear or use (either on themselves or on you) when having sex.

Invest in some classic sex texts, erotic literature or specialised books on areas that you think you might like to explore further. Read the books together, or go away for the weekend to explore new sexy ideas.

If you're trying something new for the first time and you're not sure if you really want to spend a small fortune on equipment, then improvise a bit. Think you might like bondage? Use old shirt ties, scarves and rope that are already in your home to make bonds, blindfolds and gags. Tempted by the idea of submission and domination games? Use a leather belt as a dog collar and leash.

Don't be afraid to invest in your sex life—the more you put in, the more you'll get out.

Once you have decided what you enjoy, start to splash out on a whole range of toys, games and outfits to play with. Then set aside an evening with the phone off the hook to be adventurous and creative with your new sex toys.

'Playing away' is a good prelude to introducing new ideas or techniques—a different bed from your own is always exciting and can lead to numerous new fantasy scenarios, such as tie-me-down bondage-play, or loving exploration of new positions. Treat yourself with the occasional weekend escape, an elopement to somewhere not associated with your normal life patterns (and worries).

Be inspired by the ideas in this book—try a little from different sections. Thinking of giving your partner a sensual bath? Why not follow it with a mouth massage. Got your partner all tied up? Tease them with a sexy story, whisper breathlessly into an ear. Found the perfect spot for a secluded sunny-day picnic? Why not try some tantric sex when you're out there.

Remember to be cautious when you're trying a new idea so start your sex play slowly and gently until you understand the strengths of you and your partner's desires. Also be very aware that sometimes what one of you—or perhaps both—might really need is comfortable, relaxed, cuddling, and no performance-required sex. Or you might just want an early night. Which is also OK?

Shopping for sex toys, lingerie, erotic films, books and so on creates its own momentum: the process of deciding what to buy gives you an inkling of a sexy feeling for what lies ahead; the anticipation of small packages dropping through your letter box adds to the build-up towards play time; unwrapping your surprises – both literally and figuratively – creates a delicious anticipation and shared appreciation of each other's sexuality. In this way, you build on your sex intelligence with your partner, generating life-long excitement and juiciness in your sex life.

"I love our sex dates, it keeps our relationship fresh and sexually exciting. I know that at least one evening a week we're going to spend some quality time appreciating each other and exploring the boundaries of our mutual eroticism – aside from the other times we have sex in the week. Usually, my girlfriend takes a bath first whilst I get the room ready, lighting candles and incense, setting the music, making it a sexy space. Then, she takes her time getting ready whilst I have a bath – boy, am I turned on by anticipation at this stage – and after I've dried off and maybe put on some sexy underwear myself we embark on a delicious, relaxed, sexy play time. It's the business!"

Richard, 37, Leicester.

It's All Play

Sex is too often defined as a one-way street, with kissing leading to foreplay and foreplay leading to intercourse and intercourse leading to orgasm. But what if we banish the idea of foreplay and call the whole shebang sex play instead?

Particularly in long-term relationships, it's all too easy to get into a well-worn routine where you know just how much 'foreplay' is needed before intercourse takes place and then sex starts becoming repetitive and dull.

But if you ditch the notion that foreplay is something that has to take place before intercourse, whole new erotic possibilities open up – everything becomes sex play instead, and your creative sex intelligence will find new routes to pleasure.

When did you last stop in the middle of love-making and take a break to kiss your lover's toes, or the backs of her knees, or the underside of his balls?

When it's all sex play then you're giving each other license to experiment, and open up a rich seam of juicy possibilities. It could be oral sex followed by fucking followed by masturbation followed by more oral sex and back to fucking again.

What's not to like?

Simply calling your sex date 'play-time' places it in a different category to everyday sex, giving you freedom to explore your desires in a safe space. Play is about having fun, about exploring boundaries, about enjoyment, and it has connotations of innocence – so you can leave all your hang-ups behind. Play is also (usually) about relating to other people. So in your own play-time you're giving your partner and yourself permission to be child-like and to explore each other's sexuality. You need trust and openness.

"Pleasure in sex increases substantially when we can laugh, wear costumes, let inner selves out to play, and indulge in a grown-up version of the creativity psychologists say kids engage in whenever they pick up a toy or invent the rules of a game".

Carol Queen *Exhibitionism for the Shy*

Mixing it up

By deliberately mixing up the usual sequence of kissing, arousal, foreplay, intercourse and climax we open ourselves up to other possibilities – to having separate orgasms at different stages of sex play, for instance, by different routes.

For men, this can be a liberating experience because it takes away some of their goal-oriented anxieties around sexual performance. It's also handy when intercourse is off the menu for some reason – there are so many other routes to satisfaction.

Switch the focus

Creating an atmosphere in which juicy sex play thrives means that you're less constrained by the convention of bedroom behaviour. Your sex play can stop and start with greater frequency – you can change location, change levels of arousal and anticipation more readily.

You can start in one room with one activity and move on to another way of playing elsewhere – take a break in between, change the pace, change the stimulation of all your senses. Switch from full body kissing to massage to penetration (with vibrator, dildo or penis) and then to oral sex. End with a fuck (or not, as you want...).

Indulge yourselves in the pleasures of 'heavy petting'— touching, teasing, licking, caressing, fondling, stroking, kissing and sucking. Learn to experiment with new ways of touching, from massage to masturbation.

Vary your pace: bring your partner up to a peak of excitement, hold them there for a while, and gently bring them back down a little. You can do this for hours. The arousal built up during sex play will increase the intensity of orgasm later.

If desire overwhelms you and intercourse seems inevitable, then just go ahead.

Afterwards, hold each other tight, pull apart, and go back to sex play. If you can't do this, then take a break, have a drink, change the music, start cooking supper, or whatever you feel like. But don't get dressed too much—be prepared for more later.

Plan ahead

Plan a route through the house for your lover, with different sex treats in different rooms. Blend it all together with different sensual treats at different stages. Make sure each room is fully prepared, suitably warmed up (light the fire if you have one) and candles lit.

Have the right kind of music and massage oils to hand, as well as drinks and snacks if you want them. Start with a massage in the bedroom; switch to the shower, where you can give each other a sexy rub-down (and wash off the massage oils) and oral sex; move to the kitchen, with full body kissing, tasty food treats, and a glass of wine; bring in some hot-and-cold sex toy play; finish with a prolonged climax back in the bedroom.

The permutations are as limitless as your imagination: you can start with a bath or shower together, and then retire to separate bedrooms to get dressed up for each other; meet again in the living room for a glass of champagne, where you can get into sexy dancing in your lingerie before fucking each other senseless on the sofa.

"I really relish planning our sex dates. Honestly, it gives me so much pleasure to imagine how I'm going to seduce and delight my wife. Sometimes I'll splurge our monthly sex budget and buy a new sex toy to surprise her, sometimes I'll just browse the fruit displays and imagine what I'm going to with grapes, strawberries, avocados….I like to work out how I'm going to manage the whole process, from when she walks through the door (what will I be wearing? What will she *need* at that moment? A cuddle? A glass of champagne? A neck massage?) and then take it through from there until she's lying exhausted on the floor, released and exhilarated. Of course, sometimes it doesn't always work out how I planned it. Spontaneity rules! That's also fine. I like to spin it out, though, to maximize the pleasure for both of us".

Evan, 55, London.

"We should always push ourselves a little sexually. Stay in the comfort zone all the time and you won't grow. Be willing to experiment and take a few chances. Loosen up a little, laugh a lot, drop the inhibitions and let your imagination run rampant".

Tracy Cox, *Hot Sex*.

Planning ahead for sex starts to become even more juicy once you and your partner have started to open up your sexual selves and made a commitment to trying new experiences. Sex is often more highly charged if there's a long, slow build-up – a sexy tease, whether spun out over an hour or whether planning ahead for a sex date later on in the day or the week, creates an unmistakable erotic charge which heightens the experience no end.

Planning what you're going to do for your partner, or speculating as to what they might have up their sleeve for you, is very arousing in itself. Anticipation is hot.

Make a few wicked suggestions, whisper a few seductive phrases, but don't give much away – there's nothing more thrilling than the build-up to sex play when your partner is able to anticipate your needs.

Learning to tap into your own instincts about what your partner might like – or what you know they'll be turned on by – shows a degree of sensitivity and awareness which will put you in the super-lover category and be repaid with gratitude, devotion, and as many orgasms as you can handle.

A surprise sex date can be around almost anything: it could involve something as simple as a treasure trail of sexy notes leading through the house, to where you can be found naked in the bed, bath or shower. It could involve a soft, candle-lit atmosphere with a new sex toy ready and waiting to be tried. You could be walking into a massage or a bondage session – who knows?

Some elements of surprise will keep it fresh, although once you're practised at setting up your sex dates you'll have a pretty good idea of what your partner will really go for. If you can keep being creative you will not only create many lovely, lasting memories but also you'll both keep working at the boundaries of your sexual knowledge of each other. That way, you're always expanding your repertoire and your sex lives are always growing deeper into each other.

"My husband and I very rarely make love last thing at night. Not only are we too tired by then but we often go to bed at different times. Our favourite time for sex play is the early evening. We'll take a shower, light some candles; maybe have a glass of wine, usually put on some sexy clothing. Then we have a wonderful, relaxed, multi-orgasmic play time for an hour so before dinner. We usually get dinner ready beforehand, so there's no pressure. What could be better?"

Christine, 42, Guildford.

Play-time scenarios:

- Treat him to a quickie. Wear a short skirt, stockings, suspenders, and sexy knickers or none at all. If you're not already wet with excitement when he walks through the door, then do what any street girl would do and lube yourself up beforehand. Let him know you haven't got time for foreplay – you want him now, up against the doorway, the kitchen counter, or on the sofa. Men love to be freed from the pressure of taking the traditional role in slow seduction. Let his animal masculinity rear its gorgeous head for once. Your reward will come later.

- Treat her to a deluxe pampering session. Women love to be indulged and given your full attention devoted to her needs. Start when she comes in the door; take her coat, hand her a drink, massage her shoulders...keep going with things designed to help *her* unwind, rather than to excite yourself. Give her an all-over body rub in the shower, followed by a good, long session of oral sex. Don't expect intercourse until much, much later (maybe when she's woken up from a snooze).

- Surprise him by reversing roles and nurturing his femininity. Welcome him with a bath and a gentle massage, and then dress him in your underwear. Rub his cock through your silky knickers (read Paul Theroux's novel *Blinding Light* for the ultimate literary exposition of this).

- Surprise her with a striptease. Set the mood with soft lighting, funky music, and you – all dressed up in order to get undressed. Lead her in and make sure she's comfortable before going through your strip routine (see Chapter Eight for more hints).

- Men love role reversals which mean they can be passive. Get dominant; get out your handcuffs and latex whip. And take control. Make him your sex slave for at least one sex play date. He has to do only what you tell him or he gets punished. Order him around and make sure he licks your pussy *exactly* the way you want it done – or else.

Chapter Four: Mutual Pleasures

There's no getting away from the fact that being able to masturbate your partner to orgasm, and hence both of you being able to masturbate each other, is one of the most important components of a satisfactory sex life – and juicer sex.

There used to be loads of taboos around masturbation but thankfully these are now disappearing, as a new generation of sexually-liberated couples (and singletons) have taken on board the fact that masturbation is a crucial key not just to self-knowledge, but to shared intimacy.

For most men and women, masturbation is our first natural sexual activity and one of the main ways by which we explore our own sexual responses and discover our own erotic map.

The benefits of masturbation are numerous: it gives sexual satisfaction to people without partners; it allows teenagers to have orgasms without the dangers of pregnancy or STDs; it permits partners to find sexual release when they're apart, or when one partner is ill, or not feeling like sex; it's relaxing, and helps you de-stress and sleep; it's safe sex; it's free; and, best of all, it's fun.

When sex researcher Alfred Kinsey undertook his pioneering work in the 1950s, just over 60% of women said they masturbated. By the time feminist sexologist Shere Hite carried out a similar survey in the 1970s, the figure was just over 80%. As masturbation has become more acceptable and acknowledged as positive and healthy, more and more women are doing it for themselves.

Most recently, the creators of *The Cake Report* discovered that 97% of women who responded to their questionnaire masturbated on regular basis, with an average of three to five times per week (some went as high as ten times per day!). They found that 95% of women who masturbate regularly have orgasms during partner sex.

> "It's a cause for celebration when women learn to masturbate early, and masturbate often. After our first orgasm, there's just no turning back. In one moment, we begin to understand the relationship between sexual thoughts, that feeling 'down there', our body's capability to experience pleasure, and the power of it all. Knowing what turns you on, and what gets you off, increases the likelihood that you'll engage successfully with a partner. Heck, if you don't know how to give yourself an orgasm, how can you expect your partner to take on the task?"

> Melinda Gallagher and Emily Scarlet Kramer *A Piece of Cake*

Successful creative sex play requires some useful knowledge of the female anatomy. This isn't about scoring points for knowing technical terms but about familiarising yourself with your partner's genitals so that you can give her as much pleasure, and as many orgasms, as possible. Bear in mind that the female sex organs can vary between individuals which means that a technique that was successful with a previous partner may not necessarily do the trick with a new lover. The concentration of nerve endings in the genitals is different from person to person.

Sharing masturbation is an important addition to the repertoire of couples, and to do it well it does require both partners to have come knowledge of each other's anatomy (see Her Lady Parts and His Man Bits). By familiarising yourself with your partner's genitals you'll be in a better position to give each other as much pleasure, and as many orgasms, as possible.

"A couple who can masturbate each other really skilfully can do anything else they like".

Alex Comfort *The Joy of Sex*.

Her Lady Parts

The collective name for everything you can see externally is the vulva. The fleshy mound on top of the pubic bone is the *mons pubis*. The most obvious parts after this are the outer lips or *labia majora*, usually with pubic hair on them. Between these are the inner lips, or *labia minora*, which are smooth. The Latin names—major and minor lips—can be unhelpful because both sets of lips vary widely between women and sometimes the inner lips might be bigger and more obvious than the outer lips. On arousal, both sets of lips will plump out and change to a deeper colour.

The most sensitive part of the genitals is the clitoris, hidden away under folds of skin, the clitoral hood, where her lips meet at the top. The clitoris comprises of the head, or *glans*, which is about the size of a pea and the clitoral shaft, connecting this to the rest of her nerve endings. In fact, the clitoris is not just one little nub all on its own: its part of an entire system of muscles, tissues, nerves and glands, all of which contribute to her sexy sensations. When she's stimulated, the whole area swells up and the tip of the clit becomes harder and much more sensitive. The clitoris actually has more nerve endings in it than any other organ in the human body, and it's the only part of the body whose sole function is to give sexual pleasure. For most women, direct or indirect stimulation of the clitoris is essential to orgasm.

Beneath the clitoris is the (barely discernible) urethra, through which she pees. The soft, sensitive tissues between her inner lips form the vaginal opening and beneath that, between where the labia joins together and the anus, is the perineum, also a sensitive area.

The vagina itself is a muscular canal, normally around four inches (eight centimeters) long, which expands and contracts when stimulated. The first third of the vagina is the most sensitive part, with the most nerve endings: the back two-thirds tends to be less sensitive. At the rear of the vagina is the cervix, a fleshy dome which can be sensitive to pressure.

When she's initially aroused, the first third of the vagina tends to contract and will feel tighter during intercourse. As she becomes more turned on the vagina expands and the back two-thirds often balloons outwards (for some women this takes place just before orgasm; it usually contracts again after orgasm).

Pleasing Her

Consider your hands and mouth as versatile sex tools that should be capable of turning her on and bringing her to an orgasm almost unaided by the rest of your body. Use them to stroke her skin, to stimulate her erogenous zones, and caress and excite her sex.

Be creative and playful when stimulating her, using your fingers, hands, mouth, penis, vibrator and other sex toys. Make her feel like a sex goddess.

Being able to masturbate your partner to orgasm is a skill that you'll both appreciate more than you can imagine. As you get better at giving her orgasms by hand or mouth, the more easily she'll have them. And more juicy sex will result.

Ask her how she likes to touch herself, so that you can do it the same way. Pay attention to your lover's reactions and encourage her to talk to you and let you know what she wants. Don't think that what turned on your last girlfriend will be exactly the same for your next lover.

- Don't begin to play until you've stroked, massaged and loved the rest of her body.

66

Briefly touch between her legs whilst arousing other parts of her body. Make your way slowly down to her sex with your mouth, hands and whole body. Use your hands on the belly, thighs, bum and around her pubic area.

- Squeeze and stroke until you partner is arching her back and thrusting her pelvis towards you for more direct contact. Place your hand over her pubic mound and caress her sex. Now your lover should be turned on enough so that you stimulate her further by slipping a finger into the wetness between her labia. Use slow movements as you start to play in the genital area.

- Watch her body language: if you lover is pulling away that usually means she wants a softer touch but pushing into you indicates a harder.

- Side-by-side or the 'spoons' position allows you to rest your wrist on her mound and your fingers will be in roughly the same place as hers would be if she was arousing herself.

- Another handy position for masturbating her is for you to sit upright, with her leaning back against you, which allows one hand to read her clit and the other to caress her breasts, hair and her body with your free hand.

- The clitoris usually responds best to soft, feather-light caresses but this can vary from person to person – if in doubt, ask.

- Some women are stimulated by quick movements and others by more slow ones, but whatever speed they prefer most women need a consistent, regular rhythm in order to come.

Giving her oral pleasure

To be able to give your partner fulfilling oral sex is a gift that will be repaid in sexual satisfaction for both of you. Make sure you're in a comfortable position that will allow you to sustain cunnilingus for a good long time: having your lover recline comfortably on a bed with you lying on your front between her legs is a classic. Variations on this include bending her legs

backwards towards her chest, or placing them on your shoulders. Alternatively, you can lie back on the bed, with her straddling your face, but your head will require some support. Use pillows as a positioning prop.

- Don't rush and make it clear that you've got all the time that she needs. As with finger play, work your way slowly, teasing and kissing her navel, inner thighs and *mons pubis*. Run your tongue down the crease between her pussy and thighs, brushing your lips across her labia.

- Begin with long, light strokes of your tongue up and down her vulva - don't immediately turn your attentions towards the clit. Instead, dip your tongue into her insides, and then lick up and over the clitoral hood.

- At some point she will be arching herself towards you for more direct contact with the clitoris. Give her clit a long, loving lick with your tongue or envelop it in your mouth, sucking on it like you might do on her nipples. Use your tongue to flick it gently at the same time.

- Once you get a rhythm going and she starts to build up towards a climax, keep it up until she asks you to stop. There are lots of ways to be creative with your mouth: you can just use the tip of your tongue to tantalise her clitoris, then change to the whole surface for delicious long licks.

- As well as the usual up-and-down-strokes you can move your head from side to side, or around in circles. Use your chin or nose to nuzzle her sex. If you're tongue gets tired, one technique you can use is to hold it still and move your head instead – this will give your tongue a rest!

- While you're giving pleasure with your tongue don't forget to use your hands to stroke and caress as much of her body as you can reach, especially her breasts and nipples.

- Be creative with your fingers – can you reach her G Spot at the same time?

As you become more familiar with your partner's body you'll be able to utilise your hands and fingers in all sorts of creative ways to keep her in a prolonged state of ecstasy. Stroke her g-spot while you rest your hand on her pubic area and clitoris - the pressure added by the second hand increases arousal. Or you can caress the clit with one hand whilst stroking her G-spot from the inside with the other. Try co-ordinating these movements so that both hands seem to move together towards the same point. You might use fingers or thumbs from each hand inside her, each stroking different parts of the vagina: two fingers on the G-spot, for instance, and a thumb massaging on the opposite (lower) side.

The Five Minute Orgasm

Everybody knows that most guys can bring themselves to orgasm within minutes, if they want to. Women, by contrast, need hours and hours of pampering, kissing, cuddling and 'foreplay' before they can come – or so we're led to believe. In fact, some women are perfectly capable of masturbating themselves to climax within one or two minutes, just like men. It all depends on the individual – but the burden we've put on relationships has been to assume that her orgasm 'must' come through intercourse, when it's (by now) well known that coitus only stimulates the clitoris indirectly.

Women have traditionally been afraid to stimulate themselves during sex with men because he's meant to be the one 'providing' satisfaction: a 'real man' would 'make her come'. In addition to all the pressures which this role implies, men are put in a no-win situation because the information which they've been given – that thrusting during intercourse creates female orgasms – is wrong.

The disparity between the sexual responsiveness of men and women – he's too fast, she's too slow – creates problems in many relationships, causing physical discomfort, anxiety, and unnecessary heartache. The man usually gets blamed: guys are always being told to slow down, when in fact they're biologically conditioned to come quickly. The species was designed for rapid sex: in the animal world, if you hang around too long mating, you become vulnerable to predators.

But what if we looked at this so-called problem another way around? Instead of it always being about expecting men to slow down their responses, why can't women learn to speed up sometimes – if they want to?

If both men and women accept that it's okay for women to masturbate during sex, she can bring herself to orgasm whilst having intercourse, before intercourse, after intercourse, whenever.

One particularly successful way to do this is if the woman takes control and gets on top during intercourse, then masturbates herself to orgasm. It's the main idea behind Dr Clare Hutchins' excellent book, *Five Minutes to Orgasm*. Her 'quick and easy' formula doesn't require advanced skills, multiple positions, or hours and hours of foreplay. It just requires the female partner to be able to please herself – and for a willing man to help.

"I think the most important requirement for an orgasm is reliability. Every sexual experience should be rewarded with an orgasm - we should be able to count on an orgasm every time we make love. Second, we don't want to wait all night to have one. Simple stated, it should be easy, it should be fun, and it should bring that feeling of release".

Dr Clare Hutchins *Five Minutes to Orgasm*

- The first step is for the woman to climb on top of the man, so that she has control of the action. Get your man to lie on his back, and straddle his penis. Don't be in a hurry to get him inside you. Let him enjoy being on his back and watching you. Rub yourself over him, and tease his cock into your vaginal opening. Slide it in gently when you're ready. Now you can control the amount of friction, the depth of penetration, the pace of thrusting and so on.

- The next step is to masturbate whilst you're on top of him. For some women, changing from the missionary to the female-superior position may be all that is necessary to achieve an easier orgasm. Learning how to 'ride' your man will put you in charge of your own sexual responses, rather than expecting the male to take charge of love-making.

- Most women can give themselves an orgasm pretty rapidly under the right circumstances, so by learning to masturbate yourself to orgasm whilst your partner is penetrating you, you're redefining sex as intercourse that includes an automatic orgasm for both partners. Women become less dependent on the love-making skills (or the tongue and fingers) of a man, and more in control of their own orgasmic response.

- Most men love this approach: it redefines their role, relieved from the burden of being responsible for both partner's orgasms. Also, he gets a great view of you astride his body, and he's free to watch you play with yourself in a very sex way. He also has more control over his own orgasmic response, because his body is relaxed and there's less stress and muscular tension than if he were on top of you and trying to control all the action.

"Men appreciate the fact that they don't have to wait so long for the woman to finish; they don't have to work so hard at something that should be fun; and even if they should beat the woman to orgasm, she can still finish within a reasonable amount of time by manipulating her genitals herself".

Dr Clare Hutchins, *Five Minutes to Orgasm*.

"My husband and I masturbate each other quite often so I thought that trying this technique wouldn't be a big deal - but actually I was quite surprised that when I started masturbating while on top of him it felt as though I was more deeply connecting with myself and my body - while also connecting with him. The fact that he also found it arousing was a real turn-on as well. I came pretty quickly, so then we did it again! This time he added a bit more thrusting from his position below, which was also great. Highly recommended".

Jenny, 45, London.

Female ejaculation

The ability of women to ejaculate has only recently been 'rediscovered'. The female urethral gland is very similar to the male prostrate gland, since both swell up when aroused and produce secretions. The clear alkaline fluid either squirts, flows or dribbles out during intense sexual excitement and can be mistaken for urine. The amount varies enormously—in some women it may be very small or is mixed up with semen, so as to be unnoticeable.

The G-spot is closely associated with female ejaculation, although they are not mutually dependent. Some women ejaculate on arousal, orgasm, some with the right G-spot stimulation and others only with clitoral stimulation. It's easier if your lover is on her second or third orgasm. Once she's had her first ejaculation, the second and subsequent ones should be easier. But don't make it too much of a goal, or else it becomes an unnecessary pressure.

Pleasing Him

Not a difficult task, you might think. But in fact a lot of women seem to take a pretty lazy approach to giving their man oral or manual pleasure – any attention is enough, seems to be the attitude. Lucky men that women even bother! A quick hand job to keep him quiet when she's not feeling like intercourse, and that's it. This is completely unequal, of course, and not conducive to long-term juiciness.

If you want to be treated like a goddess then it should be reciprocal in the genital-worshipping stakes. Give him as good as you want to get – treat his sensitive bits with reverence and affection, lavish praise and attention on his penis and balls, worship his *lingam* if you want to get Tantric with it. It will come back to you in spades.

Use your hair, hands, skin, mini-vibrators, boobs, silk scarves, pussy and of course mouth and lips to tease, caress and excite him. Turn his penis into your love-sexy plaything and you will be rewarded with intimacy and devotion.

His Man Bits

Most women are familiar with what the penis and balls look like externally but learning how to handle his sex is an essential skill which will enhance play for both of you.

The penis consists of a fleshy shaft containing two cylinders of spongy erectile tissue (the *corpus cavernosa*) which fill up with blood when he has an erection. Running underneath these cylinders is a third cylinder (the *corpus spongiosum*) which holds the urethra, which carries urine from the bladder. There are no bones or muscles in a penis. The smooth head of the penis is called the *glans*, and the rim around its base is known as the *corona*. The slit in the middle of the glans is the urethral opening. The glans is the male equivalent of the clitoris, although it doesn't contain as many nerve endings and is not as sensitive.

All men are born with a foreskin, which is an extension of the penile skin covering the glans. The foreskin contains dozens of nerve endings which are stimulated when it glides backwards and forwards over the head of the penis during sex. In some cultures this loose skin is removed (circumcision). Since the glans on a circumcised penis is therefore exposed at all times, it tends to be less sensitive than an uncircumcised glans.

On the underside of the glans, connecting it to the shaft, is a ridge of skin known as the frenulum. The slightly raised ridge of skin which runs from the frenulum right the way across the scrotum to the anus is called the raphe. Both the frenulum and the raphe are rich in nerve endings and can be very sensitive to touch.

The penis is connected to the pelvic cavity at its base or root. Hanging down below it is the scrotum, a loose sac of skin that holds the testes or testicles. The scrotum is designed to protect the testicles and keep them at a constant temperature (5 degrees less than body heat) for sperm production. So it will change according to circumstances: if he's cold the muscles in the scrotum contract to pull the testicles in closer to the pelvis. If he's hot, the scrotum will relax to allow his balls to hang lower. The scrotum also contracts during sex, particularly in the build-up to a climax.

The testicles are two oval glands which produce sperm and testosterone. They're very sensitive to pain and many women are squeamish about handling them for this reason. However, although a knock or tap on the testicles can be painful, firm pressure usually isn't. Most men enjoy a degree of stroking, very gentle squeezes, or tugging on the scrotum (it's why harnesses and cock-and-ball toys are so popular).

The perineum is the area between the underneath of the scrotum and the anus. As with women, this is a sensitive area which responds to stroking, licking and touching.

Some men like anal penetration during sex, others don't. Men have a pleasure centre called the prostate gland, a small, walnut-shaped gland which lies just behind the pubic bone. If stimulated during sex it can produce a very intense sensation - which is why it's sometimes called the male G-spot.

Here are some penis primers:

- Women are often surprised at how hard you can squeeze the penis. A firm, confident grip is good so don't be afraid to ask if he prefers you to hold him tighter or harder.

- Hold the base of the penis with one hand and, applying some pressure to move the penis to face away from the body, stroke upwards with the other (fingers pointing downwards), swivelling the palm of your hand over the top of his cock before stroking back down again. Make a ring with your thumb and index finger and concentrate on moving up and down on the top part of his penis (the ultra-sensitive frenulum and the head).

- Alternatively, just rotate the fingers, still in a ring around the top of the penis, until the thumb naturally lifts off.

- Keep him on the boil by caressing the penis and balls for a while and give several quick up-and-down strokes, as above, before returning to caressing (see Loving the Jade Stalk).

- With your hand on his penis, finger tips touching the scrotum, pour massage oil over your hand. Let it dribble through your fingers then take his testicles in your hands and slide them forward to touch the tip of his penis.

- Tease him further: take the root of the penis with one hand, using the other to pull the foreskin back gently. With the thumb and finger make swift strokes, for a minute of so, before returning to caressing.

- Try this. Whilst facing him, clasp your hands together as if in prayer and wrap them around his penis. Use your thumbs to caress and massage around the underside of the head and the frenulum. Take hold of the lower part of the shaft with one hand and the upper part with the other, very gently twist them backward and forwards in opposite directions. Place your palms either side of his penis, held out straight. Pretend you're trying to start a fire by the ancient stick-rubbing method. Gently roll the penis between your palms, moving rhythmically up and down the shaft as you do so.

- If you are not too heavy, sit on his chest and face his feet. Stroke his legs from the feet all the way up to his thighs, and then use each hand to stroke his perineum and balls in alternate motions, like a dog scooping out sand. You can do this for a while, then either go back down his legs and repeat or stroke up over the penis to his tummy and then repeat.

- Use a combination of these techniques, all the while trying to move smoothly from one to the next. If you've got it right, he might want to thrust his hips into the rhythm of your hands. Try not to lose your grip, but let him help you.

- Lubrication is helpful, but don't apply too much because he needs to feel some friction. Saliva can be used instead—especially if you're going to fellate him afterwards.

Loving the Jade Stalk

Tantric teachers like to string things out, and this is one technique which will have him begging for release. She takes him upwards to orgasm by whatever masturbation techniques you usually deploy, and then, sensing that he's reaching a peak, she starts on an entirely different rhythm. She stops whatever is in progress and moves to kissing, caressing or stroking his balls and penis in any way – as long as it's not actually pumping with her hand. After a short while, she gives his penis a few more really vigorous strokes or pumps with her hand (remember – holding it tight is usually good), the goes back to kissing and gentle caressing. A few seconds more, then she gives a slightly longer pump with her hand – maybe three, four, five or more strokes. Then back to gentle, not-so-frictional caressing for a brief interlude, then a really good pump with her hand for six, seven, eight or more strokes. Repeat, increasing the number of strokes between gentle caressing, until he is jelly.

Giving him oral pleasure

Some men rate blow jobs as highly as intercourse – perhaps because of their rarity value in long-term relationships. Give-and-take is the key to continuing juicy sex, so don't be shy when it comes to learning how to give a good blow-job, and of course asking him how he likes it done.

- A hand around the base or shaft, with your mouth and tongue having fun further up is a popular technique. You can enhance this by using your other hand to follow the movements of your lips up and down the shaft, with the forefinger and thumb forming a ring.

- Alternatively, as you move your hand up from the base, move your mouth down to meet it. As you raise your head, swirl your tongue across the shaft.

- Try humming whilst he's inside your mouth: the vibrations will transmit to his penis. Alternatively, hum with your lips running up and down his shaft.

- A relaxed and comfortable position for a blow job is with him on his side and you facing him, also on your side, with your head level to his genitals. Both partners can relax and it gives a new angle for you to touch and fondle him.

- During orgasm some men might want you to stop stroking immediately. Others might prefer you to carry on, though more gently, in order to maintain physical contact. Don't be afraid to ask.

- Have a mint mouthwash handy. Take a mouthful then let it dribble down his penis as you go back down on him. Mint-flavoured

edible lubricants will also create sensation, and
don't forget to lick or dribble it all over his
balls; the sensitive scrotum will appreciate the
fine sensation.

Ball games

Testicles are one of men's most neglected and
overlooked erogenous zones. Some guys even claim
they can orgasm through testicular stimulation alone.

Balls are blokes' most vulnerable and exposed body
parts and most men are not used to having them
handled by another person. If you're just starting to
play with this area, begin very gently. Once you've
mastered the right strokes and he has relaxed enough
to trust you more, he might like you to be a little
rougher - so don't be afraid to ask.

Testicles may hang low and loose in the scrotum
before arousal, but as sexual excitement intensifies
they'll move up closer to his body, with the scrotum
holding them in tight. Generally, treat testicles as you
would like your breasts to be treated: they should be
cradled, stroked, kissed, licked, and sucked.

Learn to cup his balls in your hand and then make a
circle with your thumb and index finger around the
top, and as you kiss or stroke his cock, gently tug
downwards. You can co-ordinate this with
masturbating him by pulling his balls down as your
other hand moves upwards. Stroke all the way down
his penis and then keep going, flattening your hand as

it passes over his balls. Stroke his perineum and then move back up again. Don't forget to use lubricant.

Take his balls into your mouth and use your tongue to play with them. He'll love the feeling of warm, wet, enclosure. It's often easiest to do this if you use the technique of putting your fingers around the tope of the scrotum, as described above. Try nibbling the loose skin of his sac with your lips—but don't pinch with teeth because that will hurt. Gentle scratching (with smooth not pointy nails) can also be pleasurable. The ridge which runs down the centre of the scrotum is incredibly sensitive. Explore it with your tongue, caressing his balls or cock at the same time.

After sex play is finished (not just ejaculation!), when you want to sleep, reach around and cradle his balls as you nod off—your tender touch will give him sweet, sexy dreams.

Nipples and Breasts

One of the main erogenous zones in the body, each of us is sensitive to a greater or lesser degree in the nipples and breasts. That goes for men and women. Experiment and communicate with each other, starting out cautiously and don't be afraid to show your partner where to put their hands.

Her breasts

Breasts are one of the most sensitive and sexy part of a woman's body, as we all know. If you're not yet sure what you partner likes, then ask her to show you by placing her hand over yours and stroking the area together. This can be sensuous for you both.

Different women like different techniques: squeezing, sucking, pulling, nibbling or caressing, or even a variation of all of these, plus more. Start slowly and listen to her body language as you try new techniques. Try to give the same amount of attention to each breast. Be aware that the sensitivity of her breasts and nipples might change during different stages of her menstrual cycle. Some women dislike having them touched prior to their period starting.

> "Make a dance of it, so the lovely orb is revealed with grace. If you take time to appreciate each layer, she'll appreciate you. Make it a moment. … Be playful about it and take your time".
>
> Goddard and Brungardt (Eds) *Lesbian Sex Secrets for Men*

Use your mouth, face, lips, fingers to squeeze, stroke and excite her breasts. Tease and caress, tell her how nice her breasts are when you move away to another area - before coming back for more. Kiss them before leaving and then kiss around them when you return. Always keep in touch with her breasts—an occasional touch or flick with the tongue—when you're concentrating on other areas. This will maintain arousal in that area and heighten her arousal generally.

With your thumb and forefinger in a V-shape underneath the base of her breast, stroke, using the palm of your hand, upwards and over the nipple, letting your hand go at the top of the stroke. Repeat a few times, sometimes caressing the nipple with the palm of your hand, or gently pulling it with your fingers, between strokes.

Try the five-finger caress. Start with the palm of your hand on her nipple with fingers splayed out over the breast, then gradually draw your fingertips towards the nipple, gently pulling the nipple at the end of the stroke if your partner enjoys it.

Take her nipples between your lips and suck them into your mouth, giving the tip a flick with your tongue, or a nibble with your teeth, each time. If you've made her nipples nice and wet using your mouth and tongue, then pull back and blow on them—your cooler breath with make the nerve endings tingle. Or simply slip a wet finger around and over the nipple area, pressing slightly, to increase arousal.

Some women like their nipples to be rolled between the thumb and forefinger, or pinched and pulled (gently or hard, fast or slow depending on preference). Pat attention to her body language, and ask. Spend a while teasing all around the nipple: circle the areola (the darker area which surrounds them), stroking the delicate flesh with your fingers or tongue. The area directly beneath the nipples can be super-sensitive, so take advantage of this.

If she seems to like lots of pressure, don't be afraid to use a pair of nipple clamps. Be aware, however, that women's nipples are usually much more sensitive than men's so start with a very small amount of pressure and change to suit her needs.

You can use a vibrator on your partner's breasts. Try a hand vibrator to stimulate the breast, licking and sucking one nipple, using the vibrator for the other. Try on of the small 'finger-tingler' type vibrators on her nipples, or massage her breasts and upper body with a Swedish-style model which straps on to the back of the hand (the vibrations are transmitted through your palm and fingers on to her skin).

Find out what size your partner's breasts are (discreetly look at the label on her bra) and send her little gifts of sexy lingerie—black half-cut bras or satin quarter cut bras.

Nipple clamps can provide a more intense stimulation to the nipples. Like any other kind of sex toy, it's worth going for quality. Choose metal scissors-action type clamps, linked by one or more chains, are the best kind. If they have adjustable gripping power, you can change the intensity of sensation to suit.

His nipples

Men's nipples are capable of giving considerable pleasure. Whereas some guys feel that their nipples are hot-wired to their genitals, others just don't have that same sensitivity. Don't focus for too long on his nipples if there's no immediate reaction, but don't neglect them either. Return to them at intervals and you may find that they eventually become sensitised to your touch.

Start by suck the nipples or gently pinching to find out how sensitive they are. Gently nibble, tug with your teeth or fingers, lick and tongue-flick nipples.

Try blowing on them once they're moist because the cooling sensation of your breath can create a tingling feeling. Touch him in the same way that you enjoy your nipples being touched, massaging around his nipples and kissing and fondling them. If there is less sensation in nipples, some men like them to be squeezed and pulled a little. If you think he'd like it harder don't be afraid to ask. Some guys will get hard nipples, others won't.

The G Spot

The G-spot is an elusive entity, its existence still not anatomically clarified. Some women discover that it is indeed an erogenous zone, whilst others can't locate it at all, or experience no special feelings there. But it's worth exploring to find out.

The name 'G-spot' isn't actually very helpful when it comes to finding this pleasurable area, because it's not really a spot at all, and isn't located inside the vagina. Between the vaginal opening and the clitoris lies the urethral opening, with the urethra itself surrounded by spongy erectile tissue. This is known as the urethral sponge (also called the female prostrate) and it swells during arousal. What you're actually after is a nerve mass (the urethral sponge) which can be felt *through* the upper side of the vaginal wall. Think of it as the G-zone instead.

- If you're starting out, lay your lover on her back and explore this area with your fingers - arousal will make the urethral sponge swell and easier to locate.

- Move along the top wall of the vagina until you come to a ridged section just near the front about 1–2 inches in. This ridged section is often described as having a similar 'raspy' texture to that of a cat's tongue. When it's first touched, your partner may get the feeling of needing to pee but this soon passes.

- Alternatively, with your partner on her front insert your fingers and pull down slightly towards you, pressing on the area behind the pubic bone. Either way you can press down with your other hand on the outside of her pubic mound, just above the hair-line, to help locate it.

- Once you've found the spot, circle and massage it to see how your partner reacts and what feels good. You can apply pressure and rock backwards and forwards with the rest of your hand and thumb cradling and caressing her from the outside.

- Another trick is to pressing down on the outside of her mound with one hand, whilst pressing upwards from the inside with the finger of your other hand.

- It's good to co-ordinate these movements so that both hands seem to move together towards the same point.

- Caress and rub your lover's lower belly at the same time as you caress and run inside. She might want to rock her pelvis, get into the rhythm and moan and groan to free up orgasmic energies whilst you're stroking her.

- The G-spot can also be stimulated while she's using a vibrator or masturbating herself.

- Some women prefer just to feel the G-spot sensations alone without clit touching. Try both, and gauge how she reacts.

- You can buy special G-spot vibrators, usually with a curved tip which bends around to try and touch the G-spot from the inside. However, the most important stimulus for the G-spot is pressure rather than vibration. Curved dildos are better for this, since the female can move against it whilst the dildo stays in place.

G-spot orgasm might or not might happen. Don't fret either way, just enjoy! If an orgasm is approaching, it's possible that a lighter touch will encourage the orgasm to arrive fully. You both need to communicate to find out what your partner needs. The best positions in penetrative intercourse to achieve G-spot stimulation in your partner is to use the rear entry position, or to have your lover on top of you.

The Prostate

The male prostate is a small, walnut-shaped gland lying just beneath the bladder behind the pubic bone. Its purpose is to produce ejaculatory fluid but it is also a source of intense pleasure for men, which is why it's sometimes called the male G-spot. Stimulating the prostate during oral sex or masturbation can give your partner an explosively intense orgasm. Some men can climax from this kind of stimulation alone, producing a steady stream of ejaculate rather than sudden spurts.

- Start by massaging his lower back, buttocks and thighs to loosen up the whole area.

- Turn him over, lubricate his genitals, and give them some loving rubbing until he is highly aroused, taking him almost to orgasm before backing off.

- First, stimulate the prostate externally, massaging the perineum area between his balls and his anus by pressing, and circle with your fingers. Vibrate with the flat of your hand or the knuckles of your fist pressed up against this area to help stimulate and loosen him up.

- Using plenty of lube, massage and circle the anus and then very gently insert your finger. His sphincter muscles will probably tense up, in which case you can pause briefly and then wiggle or rock your finger in small movements until he relaxes enough to let it in further.

- When it's inside a couple of inches, crook the finger and stroke against the tissues in roughly the 12 o'clock position. You should be able to feel a round, firm spongy gland. Try different strokes or vibrations to discover which is the most pleasurable.

- You can stimulate the prostate and penis in one coordinated movement: Stroke upwards with the finger that's inside him whilst at the same time stroking downwards on his penis, as if your fingers and hand are going to meet, continuing back downwards (finger) and upwards (hand) on the reverse stroke.

- A Tantric technique to stop him climaxing is to press firmly (rather than stroke) on the prostate as a climax approaches. Then, relax totally for a while before starting again. As he reaches peak after peak his orgasms will blend into one continuously ecstatic flow.

Chapter Five: Juicy Intercourse

Intercourse should come naturally to us as a species – after all, it's how we reproduce and propagate our own kind. It is one of our primary acts, but being such as powerful act also means that it carries layer upon layer of cultural significance. This helps determine who you do it with, how you do it, what meaning you give to the act itself, and all the other emotional, spiritual, political and physical preconceptions you bring into the bedroom with you.

Does this matter? On one level, emphatically no – two people, madly in lust, hurriedly tearing off each other's clothes to passionately make love because their instincts and emotions tell them that they must have intercourse with this person NOW is a marvellous, erotic, life-affirming act.

But on another level, yes it is important – because how you make love with your partner and how you interact together in bed is key in terms building the intimacy, trust, and loving energy that flows between you.

Having good, juicy intercourse together is a skill. It involves communications, empathy, and sexual intelligence. It can just happen naturally and fluidly, and carry on doing so. But often it runs into the rocks as boredom, frustration, and poor communication scupper your chances of enthusiastic bonking.

It doesn't have to be that way. For instance, hopefully by now you will have picked up enough tips to realise that intercourse is not always the main course – it could be the starter, it could be the final course. Adding spice, variety and juicy sex dates to your love life will keep your relationship fresh and stimulating.

Again, once you and your partner have learned to masturbate each other to your mutual satisfaction then you're both liberated to enjoy the classic sex act in all its wondrous manifestations, including the thousands of variants that humans have come up with to make it even more enjoyable still. Sometimes these might involve fingers, dildos, mouths, vibrators, grapes, harnesses, straps, ice cream, hands, feet, paddles, cock rings, lubricants and many other objects (including lingerie and bedroom wear) besides.

> "It's God's fault that couples have so many problems with intercourse. If he really wanted women to enjoy it, he would have out the clitoris *inside* the vagina. I mean, what was he thinking? The only sex organ in the body designed exclusively for sexual pleasure and it's stuck right up there in penile no-man's land. This simple design fault has caused no end of problems".

Tracey Cox *Hot Sex*.

Classic acts

The conventional, timeless classic position for intercourse is for the man to be on top as the active partner, thrusting in and out with his penis whilst the woman lies underneath and 'receives' him as the passive partner.

Nothing wrong, of course, with the good old 'missionary position' in the right time and place – but actually there is a lot wrong with it as a general model for couples' sex relations.

Firstly, it's very unlikely to bring her to orgasm and secondly it's a very unequal position: he's mostly active, she's largely passive, and this can set up a situation whereby this becomes the model for your sexual interactions generally. Often, he gets tired of always being the active or initiating partner (and of having to 'do all the work') and she gets bored because she's uninvolved and not bringing much to the party. This is an extreme example, of course, and not many couples fall into this range. But there can be elements of this which will permeate other aspects of your sex lives.

Other complications include the fact that as the active partner the male may have to take on the responsibility for their orgasms – for both of them! He's mean to 'make her come' and at the same time prevent himself coming and yet he's in a position (the missionary) which is contra-indicated for either of these events happening. It's not easy for her to come, but it is easy for him.

Not surprisingly this can lead to anxiety, increased pressure on him, and the development of issues such as 'premature ejaculation' (I put that in inverted commas deliberately. How can it be premature when the position is designed to make it happen as quickly as possible?).

Besides this, there's another big issue: with men cast in the active role, they can miss out big time on the joys of being passive – of learning to receive, to open up to their own vulnerability, and to being loved and cared for. Conversely, the female partner is denied the opportunity to enjoy being in control, of taking charge of the event, and of being an active giver.

This is why men often adore being tied down and made love to: giving into to passivity and receiving love is not always a role model they've been taught. It's also why many couples nowadays enjoy sex games and role-playing, perhaps spiced up with some fantasy sex or BDSM.

Of course there are often occasions when male testosterone and his natural instincts will put him in the driving seat (so to speak) and he'll take over the active role from start to finish. That's fine too – but just remember that she needs her orgasm somewhere en route, or else we're pretty much in caveman territory as regards mutual obligation and respect. And it's also *her* responsibility to facilitate this in the easiest possible way for him, either by showing him beforehand or telling him at the time – or doing it herself. Otherwise, again, it's not an equal relationship.

Whilst women might moan about a lack of orgasms in 'straight' intercourse positions, men are just as likely to resent the lack of enthusiasm or participation on her part.

The answer – as we saw earlier – is for you both not to rely on intercourse for her to orgasm. And for her to then properly *enjoy* being an active participant in sex – because, after all, she's going to be guaranteed of getting her orgasm (or orgasms even), usually beforehand (or by hand...).

> "The factor that most determines whether or not you'll enjoy intercourse is your ability to be an active participant rather than a passive one. Intercourse is an exchange of energy, spirit, passion and love. It isn't intended to be simple tolerated. The act commands respect, both for you and your partner. Lying there like a bump on a log whilst he thrusts himself in and out of you is not a demonstration of respect, spirit, passion, or love."

Lou Paget *How to Be a Great Lover.*

Exploring Positions

There are hundreds of different positions in which to have intercourse, although most are variations on half-a-dozen or so old favourites. Different positions will produce different kinds of stimulation for each partner. Some will give you both more skin-to-skin contact, whilst others are more suitable for stimulating each other manually or with sex toys at the same time.

- Don't get stuck in a routine. Talk about what you'd like to try, experiment once in a while with variations on your regular pattern of penetrative sex.

- Don't expect to repeat every position: although some will become part of your repertoire there will be others that you don't enjoy so much which will be discarded as a one-off bit of fun.

- Some positions will suit particular occasions, or moods, or, more practically, people of certain shapes, heights.

- A sense of humour is an asset when playing with new positions so be prepared to forego embarrassment and you won't go too far wrong.

- Try to acquire the knack of moving together fluidly between positions so that you can use them in creative series.

- Don't confuse athleticism with eroticism—simply manipulating your partner through a series of manoeuvres isn't sexy. But moving gracefully from one passionate clinch to another can keep you both in a state of continual ecstasy.

- Whatever position you're in, don't forget to use the rest of your body (including your mouth, lips, hair, hands, and feet) to stimulate your partner. Don't let your body parts lie there idle (unless you're enjoying being passive).

"Whatever you do, do it with passion. Both of you will get a lot more out of all that humping and grinding if you thrust your hips up to meet each other's, grab bottoms and pull them closer to you, run your hands up and down backs, arms and backs of thighs and lick or bite the closest thing to your mouths. Go for it. Make so much noise, your neighbours consider double-glazing their windows".

Tracey Cox *Hot Sex*.

Him on Top

In the basic 'missionary position' the woman lies on her back with her legs apart and the man lies on top. This traditional position is one of the most frequently-used by couples of all ages. It's a satisfyingly comfortable position that gives you both plenty of skin to skin sensations and intimate, face to face kissing, talking and eye contact. For her it can be enjoyably passive—he is the more active partner in this position—and her hands are free to caress his body. It's easier for her to reach her clitoris than it is for him to do so. For him it feels good because he can control the depth, angle and pace of penetration. She can move beneath him to increase his pleasure.

There are light variations on this basics position. The woman can put her legs on her partner's shoulders for increased penetration, tilting the legs up or down to a greater or lesser degree dependent upon flexibility. Alternatively, the man might lift legs of his lover folding the knees to her breasts, and with the soles of her feet resting on his chest; he can penetrate deeply, holding the soles of her feet as he moves. Try putting a couple of pillows or cushions underneath her, which will tilt her pelvis upwards and create different sensations.

Her on Top

The opposite of the missionary position and equally as popular. The man lies on his back and the women sits or lies facing him. In this position, the man can be lying on his back or sitting (on the floor or on a chair).

Women like this position because she can control how deep he goes inside her vagina and equally tease him to vary the levels of his arousal. There are numerous ways for her to play including rubbing her labia against the shaft of his penis, slipping his penis in and out of her vagina, or brushing her breasts against him.

It's a great position for clitoral contact—both of you can reach out to caress the other, or use a vibrator. His hands are also free to roam over her body and caress her breasts. Her hands are free to stroke his chest or reach around to touch his balls, or to stimulate her own breasts. You can both kiss each all over your upper bodies. Men like this position because not only are they mostly passive but it's also great to be able to watch her in action.

As a variation, she can squat on her feet (rather than resting on her knees) which will give her greater mobility to twist about on top of him. She can swivel all the way round, until she's facing away from him. Again, you might find that you can both move into different positions, such as side-to-side position or rear-entry, from this one position.

Taking it from behind

Rear entry (or 'doggy style') positions usually involve the women on her hands and knees, with the man penetrating her from behind either standing, kneeling or with one foot on the floor and the other kneeling. Because there's no eye contact, both of you can fantasize about who you're having sex with.

Rear entry positions present the woman in a very submissive position while the man dominates. This position increases the depth of penetration, and the angle of the penis should mean that it's stimulating the front wall of the vagina and her G-spot. He is able reach to stimulate her breasts or clitoris whilst inside her, and she can also easily play with his balls or her clitoris. Because her breasts will be hanging downwards, the nipples will be more sensitive because of the increased blood flow. His whole groin area will have lots of stimulating contact with her bottom. A downside to this position is that the intense sensitivity can cause him to have an orgasm sooner than desired.

The angle of penetration can be varied by changing positions. She might have her elbows on the pillows, she can lie face down on the bed with her legs apart, or she could kneel on the floor bending over the edge of the bed (or sofa or office desk). To give more reach he can raise one leg whilst penetrating her.

Side-by-side

With the woman lying on her side, the man enters her from behind —a position usually known as 'spoons'.

With her bottom snuggled into his crotch and his arms holding her tight, this is a very cosy, comfortable position. It's perfect for lazy, relaxed sex, as both partners can enjoy themselves without having to work too hard at it. She can move her bottom invitingly against him or swivel her hips in rhythm. He can kiss the nape of her neck, and fondle her all over. Her reach is more limited, although she should be able to caress his balls or perineum. Either partner can stimulate her breasts and clitoris. Because it's such a relaxed position it's easy for him to slow down or rest to control his orgasm. This is a good position for pregnant women or if one partner is heavier than the other.

Try side-by-side facing each other, with your legs resting one on top of the other. This will give more face to face contact, although penetration won't be quite so full. Or you can swivel from here into an X-position, with your heads at opposite ends of the bed and your legs in a scissors shape. You can either fondle each other's genitals during intercourse or simply hold hands and let your bodies do the rest. This can be performed in either a lying-down or sitting position.

Standing up

In standing sex the woman usually leans back against a wall or other surface whilst the man penetrates her. However, you really need to be of compatible heights for him to be able to insert his penis comfortably or this position just won't work. Alternatively, the shorter partner will have to use some props (a box, a step, or maybe she can wear high heels) to even out the difference. If you can get this right, it's a terrific position for daring, naughty sex because you can perform anywhere (clothes and laws permitting). It's the position most often associated with lustful, spontaneous 'quickies', when passion catches you far away from the bedroom in a public or semi-public place. However, having sex standing up can be tiring and it's not for everyone.

A variation is for him to stand upright with his back to the wall with her legs around his waist whilst he holds her up (this takes a strong man and/or much lighter woman in order to work). Alternatively she might face away from him, holding on to the wall or the furniture, whilst he penetrates her from behind. This variation lets him reach around to her clitoris or breasts.

"Another sexual position myth that I'd like to explode, and that'll also help revolutionise your lovemaking, is that there's nothing stopping you from having a break in the middle of sex. We have this restrictive and inhibiting belief that once we start penetration we shouldn't stop until we've reached climax. Nothing could be further from the truth! In fact, stopping and resting during your sexual experience can actually heighten your sexual pleasure. I've known couples who stop and pour themselves a glass of wine, or even make a cup of tea and share some finger foods in the middle of sex. They might share some sexy banter or a loving cuddle or simply lie back for a few moments to re-energize".

Pam Spurr *Sensational Sex.*

Chapter Six: Tantric Love and the Ancient Sexual Arts

Every culture in history has had its own spin on sex, with some of the better known ones being the Indian texts of the *Kama Sutra*, the ancient Arabic works translated as *The Perfumed Garden*, and the Oriental belief systems of the Tao and Tantra.

All these philosophies and sexual texts have something to offer those of us in search of more, better, juicier sex today.

The best approach is to try a lucky dip (as with everything else in this book). Set yourselves up for a sex date with your partner, call it what you wish – Oriental night, Tantric night, Kama Sutra night – and create as much of an atmosphere as you're able to which will reflect the theme: Indian scarves draped over lampshades, maybe, to create a soft light, accompanied by some heady Eastern scents (patchouli is an old favourite for hippy types). Make sure you're wearing loose, comfortable clothing: sarongs, harem pants, or silk pyjamas are all good.

All these different ways of making love have some kind of spiritual element. It doesn't matter whether or not this means anything to you, in some cases it's easy enough to simply take the techniques and apply them to your own lovemaking. But on the other hand it would be a shame if the spiritual side passes you by entirely – you may find that it adds another dimension not just to your sex life but to also to the emotional depth of your encounters and to the passion in your relationship.

An oriental or exotic sex date can be enormously fun-filled and joyous event which also has the power to enrich and deepen your love life in numerous ways. You can bring in an element of massage, dance, self-loving, and sex talk which will overlap with your other sex dates and feed the new sexual energy growing between you. It can provide you with an entirely new direction on its own, leading both of you into states of ecstasy you've never experienced previously. At the very least, it will help shift your focus and nudge you towards a much more open, communicative and loving relationship.

> "The sexual ecstasy of a woman has a very high value. It is a magical, healing force. When she has been well loved, sexually fulfilled, she herself becomes a goddess with magical powers – radiating love, devotion, caring, gratitude, happiness".

> Margot Anand *Sexual Ecstasy*.

Taoism

This is an ancient Chinese philosophy which taught that the art of love-making should be studied and practised as much as possible, encouraging new techniques in order to surprise and please a partner.

At the heart of Taoism is the idea of a life force, or *chi*, which runs through all living beings, including us. This life force travels through meridians or energy channels in our bodies – it's the same energy flow which is central to Eastern practices such as tai chi, acupuncture or reflexology.

According to the Tao, at the heart of the spirit body is three energy centres: the uppermost is in your head (controlling the intellect), the middle one is behind your breastbone (controlling emotions) and the lowest one is located in your belly (controlling physical desires).

A Taoist approach to sex involves becoming aware of these energy centres during lovemaking in order to achieve harmony and balance between them – which then promotes increased energy flow and greater vitality. By harnessing 'chi' (your sexual energy) you intensify the experience by mentally directing it around and through you and your partner's bodies.

Sexual essence

According to the Tao for both men and women sexual essence is an important 'storage battery' for our vital energy. The essential difference between the sexual nature of man and woman is in the nature of male and female orgasm. When a man ejaculates, he ejects his semen-essence from his body. When a woman reaches orgasm, she too 'ejaculates' all sorts of sexual secretions internally, but these are retained within her body.

In conventional sexual relations, a man ejaculates every time he has intercourse, regardless of his own age or condition. From the Taoist perspective, this gradually robs him of his primary source of vitality and immunity leaving him weak and vulnerable to disease and shortening his life span. However, the love-juices of a woman are considered directly beneficial to man's health and this female 'nectar' can either be absorbed through the tongue, or the skin of the penis.

Hence, the woman is central to the art of making love, say the Taoists. She is brought to orgasm before any orgasm by the man is considered. And for the man, ejaculation should be reserved for special occasions.

So the woman enjoys complete unrestricted sexual pleasure in exchange for a measure of her abundant supplies of life-prolonging essence and energy. In order to fully satisfy his partner in bed, as well as nurture rather than deplete his essence and energy, a man must learn to prolong the act as long, and resume it as often, as is necessary for his partner to experience complete satisfaction.

You don't have to accept all of Taoism in order to incorporate some of these ideas into your own love-making and make it more enjoyable. For example, here are some Taoist ideas which will allow the man's penis to absorb as much of the woman's juice as possible – which we think is, in general, a very good idea.

- He can thrust deep inside her but withdraw slowly to drag out some of the goodness that will be absorbed through his skin.

- To control ejaculation, stimulate the entrance of the vagina with three shallow thrusts, then take two deep thrusts. Follow this with three more shallow thrusts near the entrance, then two deep thrusts again. After the first ten, pull out and rest briefly before continuing the same pattern. You can thrust deep and rhythmically, benefiting from the juices but without coming, but this requires a good knowledge and practice of the special exercises required to prevent ejaculation.

- As the man nears climax he should squeeze his PC muscles, stopping the sexual charge from being released. Instead, concentrate on sending the chi energy up your spine to your brain, holding your breathe as you do so and then releasing it slowly whilst still maintaining the squeeze. Repeat several times. Practicing contracting the perineum muscles whilst not having sex will help strengthen them for this technique.

- Vigorous massage of a man's feet and toes will stimulate energy to travel to the associated organs. The liver, which controls and releases the extra supplies of blood require to engorge the penis, is directly stimulated by foot massage. Therefore regular stretching, massaging, flexing and acupressure of the feet and toes, when adopted as a daily exercise, help promote and maintain overall male sexual vitality.

'Over time you train yourself to be sensitive to the dynamic balance of love and desire, holding and releasing, starting and stopping, foreplay and fucking, stroking and licking, kissing and sucking, pushing and pulling, hardness and softness, activity and passivity, giving and receiving, tension and relaxation, thrusting hard and merely wiggling about—Yin and Yang'.

The Barefoot Doctor's Handbook for Modern Lovers.

The Tantric Way

Central to the idea of Tantra is the energy-body, with seven energy centres known as chakras which run down the length of your body, from the crown chakra at the top of the head to the root chakra located at your perineum. Sexual energy circulates between the chakras along well-defined pathways.

One of the central ideas behind Tantra (like Taoism) is that by using breathing, you can redistribute your energy from your genitals throughout your body, leading to a more intimate connection with your partner.

Although the ultimate goal may be orgasm, the importance lies in the build up of sensation and arousal over time. This mostly involves very slow love-making, plenty of eye contact, synchronised breathing, and sensual touching, concentrating on the flow of energy between you. When eventually the woman reaches orgasm, it will be longer and fuller because she is fully relaxed and sensitised. Like Taoist sex, Tantric sex concentrates on servicing the needs of the woman to the benefit of both partners.

> "Instead of sex being a purely physical experience – a kind of genital sneeze – it becomes a way of opening your heart and mind to the purest forms of love and unity. You become inspired by greater levels of passion and pleasure than you may have thought possible".

Val Sampson *Tantra: The Art of Mind-Blowing Sex.*

Tantric warm-ups

To 'wake up' your body, stand with legs apart at hip-width, and shake yourself all over. This will increase sensitivity throughout your body. You and your partner can then start to share your energy using the simple practice of breathing and rocking.

- Sit on the floor facing your partner. The woman can either sit on his lap or kneel between his crossed legs with his legs wrapped around her.

- With closed eyes, start to concentrate on your breathing. When you exhale, your partner should inhale.

- Continue to breath and, looking into your partners eyes, begin to rock back and forth in harmony with your partner. Continue to make eye contact and concentrate on your breathing as you rock.

- Gradually you will both find yourselves in the same state of relaxation and will have made a deeper connection with each other.

The Heart Salutation

The heart salutation is an important Tantric tradition because it signals a break with the mundane, everyday world and an acknowledgement that you're moving into different territory – a sacred sexual space, if you like. It also honours the sex god and goddess within each of you.

If you've travelled in Asia you're probably familiar with the *namaste* greeting, which is widely used as a way of saying 'hello'. Its literal meaning is 'the God in me salutes the God in you' and this Tantric version harks back to that acknowledgement of each others' divine essence – this case, divine sexual essence.

You might feel a bit self-conscious trying this out at first, but with time – and further sex dates – it will become part of your routine and will help put you in a Tantric frame of mind.

- Sit facing your partner, either naked or wearing a loose robe or sarong, depending on what you're comfortable with.

- Gaze into each other's eyes softly for a few minutes, then inhale and bring your hands together as if in prayer, with your thumbs resting against your chest.

- Close your eyes and exhale, leaning forwards from the waist as you do so. Lean forward until your foreheads touch. Hold this connection, feeling the energy flow between you.

- Inhale, straighten up and look into your partner's eyes.

- At this point, you can either just say 'namaste' or you can go further and add whatever you like that recognises your partner. For instance: "[partner's name], I honour the sex god/goddess within you". As your connection with your partner deepens through the exercises in this book, you will realize the truth of this.

- Take your time – a good *namaste* connection is like foreplay.

Going deeper

By now, you may be starting to become aroused, but continue to focus on the devotionally erotic aspects of your touching. Take turns at giving each other a

113

steamy bath or use other the massage techniques. You should both start becoming more relaxed and begin to feel a slow build up or erotic anticipation. Focus on the less obvious erogenous zones, such as massaging an ear with your fingertips, stroking the thigh, or running your fingers over the arch of the foot before massaging the toes. Move your touch gently and maintain as much eye contact as possible. If you want to turn the heat up then do.

Move to more direct genital stimulation. Take your partner to the maximum arousal but don't climax. Tantric sex uses the technique of reaching maximum arousal and then bringing down the tempo. This is repeated over some time. Take a break to calm yourself down. Stop and focus on your breathing, maybe just for a couple of minutes. When you finally climax it will be longer and more pleasurable because you will have fully sensitised your bodies.

There are five main Tantric positions: woman on top; man on top; side to side, facing each other; seated face-to-face.

It also teaches five basic oral sex positions: The man stands, squats or is seated, and the woman is kneeling or seated, and she fellates him; the woman is standing, squatting or seated over the man, with her labia within reach of his mouth; a '69' position with the man on top; a '69' position with the woman on top; the man lies or sits, with the woman lying, sitting or squatting above him, facing towards his feet.

Tantric traditions tend to favour a specific number of penetrative strokes of one kind followed by a specific number of another kind: for instance, ten slow up-and-downs, followed by five real quick thrusts, then ten more slow ones. You don't have to count the strokes, but changing the tempo is a good way to vary sensations and keep your partner on edge.

Because of the different arousal rates of men and women, you should always begin by using the above positions to stimulate the woman. Experiment until you find what suits you both, but generally, to begin, those in which he gives her oral–genital stimulation are best.

Holding the base chakra

This Tantric practice is a wonderful way of connecting with your partner's *muladhara*, or base chakra (located at the perineum). Lie down on your backs side by side but facing in opposite directions – with your feet at your partner's head and vice-versa. Place your hand on your partner's genitals, resting it lightly to begin with – you can lift one leg if that makes it easier, but try and stay as relaxed as possible.

Feel the energy moving up your body as you breathe – after a while you can alternate periods of stillness with caressing your partner's genitals, sensing the energy rising as they get more excited – but keep it at a slow, gentle level. You will find you can both go on like this for a long time very pleasurably, stroking and caressing his *lingam* (penis) and her *yoni* (vagina). His hand will fall naturally with the thumb able to enter her and caress her g-spot whilst his other fingers are spread out across her mound. After having aroused her sufficiently, he can move his thumb out and bring her to a climax whilst stimulating her clitoris. She can meanwhile keep stroking his genital area, but pausing every so often to feel the energy.

"This is an exercise to feel the energy rising from the base chakra up through the pelvic chakra and beyond. Try to feel the warmth your lover's hand generates in and through your genitals. If during this exercise either person becomes aroused to the point of orgasm then that's all right. Because we are orgasm-oriented in the west it may take a while to learn to focus on the energy rather than the sexual/spiritual experience".

Richard Craze *Tantric Sexuality*.

"I loved this Tantric position straight away. Having already given my partner a Tantric massage and an orgasm, it was great to lie there and just gently play and stimulate her whilst enjoying the way she was holding and stroking my cock. Every time I breathed in and out I could feel the energy moving up my body. I think we both felt ourselves to be in a very non-linear space: there was no beginning or end; we could have gone on for hours like this without rising to a climax, but just staying in a state of glorious sexual excitement. Eventually I decided to change to pace with my fingers and fairly quickly she was having another massive orgasm. I decided I wanted her to do the same to me, which she did, and pretty soon after that I felt I needed to bring us together and just fuck, having the most amazing climax in the process".

Ethan, 28, London.

The Tantric energy flow

Like Taoism, many Tantra teachers believe that the male should absorb as much of the female's precious vaginal fluids as possible, orally and through his skin, whilst conserving his own semen. Whilst the woman's fluids are her energy and she can share these with her partner, the belief holds that the man will lose all his energy if he ejaculates.

Here are some ways you can incorporate Tantric techniques:

- When you are both ready to have penetrative sex, the male partner should try not to thrust at all because he must concentrate on holding back, using his PC muscles to conserve his energy for longer lasting sex play.

- You can move together into the sitting position, him cross-legged with her facing him, resting on her calves in a sort of kneeling position. From here he can enter her and the woman should use the thighs to control movement up and down. You can continue to caress and kiss and, of course, retain eye contract.

- From here you can move into man-on-top positions (with her legs out straight or back over her head) and then into a side-by-side position facing each other, and then a side-by-side position with her back to him.

- Learn to move gracefully between these positions, like a spiritual dance. This will come naturally to some couples but might require practice for others. All the while you should be concentrating on your breathing, each breath blending into and absorbing that of your partner's breath.

- If the man needs to withhold orgasm to continue to concentrating on spiritual touching, there is a south Indian Tantric trick: grasp the penis at its root (the perineum) and, pressing hard, expel air slowly through the

nose, at the same time contracting the anal
muscles, drawing them inward and upward.

Tantric tongues

Some Tantric teachers believe that the tongue is one
of the most important organs in the body, and that by
keeping the tip of your tongue pressed up against the
roof of your mouth you complete the energy flow
around your internal circuits – in fact, some even
suggest that you should keep your tongue in this
position *all day* in order to increase the flow of energy.

You probably don't want to go that far. But we can
incorporate some ideas on Tantric 'tongue work'
during lovemaking. This involves placing your tongue
directly on your lover's body – on their lips, genitals,
ears, neck, feet, nipples or anywhere else – in order to
give and receive sexual energy.

Explore your lover's mouth with your tongue, explore
their genitals, and explore the whole of their body.
Use your tongue skilfully to create artful loving, say
the Tantric.

"Start by placing your tongue gently on the side of your lover's neck. Now, very slowly, move your tongue, dragging its tip across your lover's skin, noticing how it affects the energy in his or her body. After using your tongue gently in this way, begin to press your tongue more forcefully into your lover's neck, as if you were trying to reach your lover's heart with your tongue. Keep going on other parts of your lover's body, sensing how it affects their mood and energy flows".

David Deida *The Enlightened Sex Manual.*

The Kama Sutra

This is one of the best known of the ancient sex manuals, renowned for its explicit descriptions of intercourse positions. The original is in fact much more than that. Written around the 4th century AD by the nobleman Vatsyanana, it was etiquette manual for Indians of similar rank and includes topics seducing a lover, selecting a wife, and running a household. However, there is still much that translates well to modern sexual modes.

The five senses

'Kama' means the 'enjoyment of appropriate objects by the five senses of hearing, feeling, seeing, tasting and smelling, assisted by the mind together with the soul'. 'Sutra' is a precept or aphorism. The Kama Sutra follows the Tantric tradition of viewing the human body as a temple, and the sex act as a sacred sacrament to help you achieve enlightenment. The books also includes topics such as choosing aphrodisiacs, applying scent, and providing a 'pleasure room' strewn with flowers to put you in the right frame of mind.

As well as the famous 'positions', The Kama Sutra acknowledges the power of a range of sex play activities, including embracing, kissing, 'scratching with nails', and biting.

There are many ways to embrace your lover, according to the Kama Sutra. One such is the *twining of the creeper* where a woman clings to a man like a creeper on a tree: he bends his heads towards her, she make the sound of 'sut sut' and looks lovingly towards him, whilst maintaining the embrace. The *embracing of the forehead* occurs when one lover touches the other at the mouth, the eyes and the forehead.

The Kama Sutra describes many kind of kissing. This includes the *bent kiss* where the heads of the two lovers are bent together to kiss. The *turned kiss* occurs when one lover turns the face of the other by holding the head and the chin and kisses it. A *pressed kiss* is one in which the lower lip is pressed with much more force. The *greatly pressed kiss* requires on lover o hold the other's lower lip, caressing it with the tongue, and kissing the lips very hard.

All places that can be kissed can also be bitten but without breaking the skin. These range from hard to soft. When biting is done using all the teeth, it is known as *line of jewels*. The *swollen bite* sees the skin pressed down on both sides. Considered for those of intense passion, the *biting of a boar* results in rows of marks near to one another, with intervals of red skin, impressed on the breast and shoulders.

The Karmic positions

The Karma Sutra is famous for offering lots of positions, so here are a few of the most popular.

- In *The Yawning Position* he kneels down, she lies on her back with her legs stretched outside either side of his waist. It's visually very erotic for the man, and he can also easily reach her clit or breasts. It doesn't allow for deep penetration so it's comfortable for her if his penis is big.

- *The Position of the Wife of Indra* requires that the woman lies on her back with both her legs drawn back to her chest. He kneels to penetrate her, whilst her feet are resting on his abdomen. This position is good for deep penetration, so works well for the less well-hung or during the advanced stages of sex when her vagina expands. He can also reach her clit, and she can easily tense her vaginal muscles as she builds up towards orgasm.

- In *The Mare's position*, the man lies down or sits; she mounts him facing towards his feet. It's a good position for her to squeeze his penis with her vaginal muscles, and she can also stimulate her clit or his balls or both at the same time. He can caress and nibble her arms and shoulders, and also reach her breasts or clitoris.

- *The Congress of a Cow* requires both partners standing up, she bends over, supporting herself with her hands on the floor, and he penetrates her from behind. This is a deep penetration position that also gains an erotic charge from being quite animalistic. He controls the speed and depth of thrusts and can move her against his body by holding her waist or hips. For both partners it provides the stimulation of his body moving against her buttocks, and he can also reach her breasts or clit.

- In *The Suspended Congress*, he leans back against a wall, she holds on to his neck and he lifts her by the buttocks or thighs. Good for a 'quickie' or passionate tryst outside of the bedroom, but he will need to be strong or she needs to be lightweight for it to work.

Chapter Seven: Juicy massages

Massage is a wonderful way of connecting with your partner and creating more juicy play time.

There are dozens of different styles of massage. But don't worry if you don't know any of these techniques - simply offering massage and giving love with the movement of your warm, oiled hands over your partner's body is enough to generate positive energy in your relationship.

Many massages (such as Tantric) are explicitly sexual, and there's no denying the erotic potential of the sensual massage environment, nakedness, warm oil, and skin-on-skin contact. This erotic potential is also enhanced by the fact that it's a gift from one of you to the other – and therefore it's also a gift to your relationship. The energy that you put in will be returned to you in the form of a warmer, sexier relationship.

Massage is also very helpful in re-connecting and building trust with your partner if you have spent a period being apart emotionally or physically. A long, slow, gentle massage with warm oil and firm hands is a soothing, healing experience. It's also a good way of getting to know your partner's body or re-discovering it, and a way to re-kindle your love and affection for each other.

There may be times when massage doesn't lead to sex – it can simply be a gift to your partner, without expectation of getting something back. Sometimes you just need to leave him or her lying blissfully relaxed under a warm towel and quietly exit the room. So don't always expect your massage to be immediately reciprocated.

> "There are no special tricks to massage – no hours of practicing weird techniques – no tedious new vocabulary to learn. With a warm quiet place and a bottle of scented oil you can spread pleasure over every inch of your partner's body. You don't need a lot of money or a room full of special equipment to do this. People were massaging each other before money or special equipment existed. And you don't need an intensive course in anatomy to lay your hands on another human being".
>
> Gordon Inkeles and Murray Todris *The Art of Sensual Massage*.

The massage environment

You will hopefully already have set up your bedroom so that it's more conducive to juicy sex, with sensual furnishings and soft lighting, so not much more is needed apart from maybe some relaxing music and incense.

Most important is where you're going to give and receive massage. Most beds are too soft for massage and you're better off on the floor, either using an airbed, foam cushion or folded blankets. Cover whatever you're using with old towels.

Some kinds of massage (nuru massage, for instance), will require other items.

Massage tables

If possible I recommend investing in a massage table: there are plenty of good quality folding massage tables available on the internet for around £150, which isn't a great deal of money considering how much use you will get from it over the years - consider it as a long-term investment in your relationship – and your sex life!.

Try www.massagewarehouse.co.uk or
http://massagetablestore.com

Massage oils are also widely available, or you can simply use baby oil or light household oils such as sunflower, grape seed or soya oil. Some people swear by olive oil, while others find it too thick. If your massage flows into a genital massage, switch to a water-based lubricant if you're going to be putting it directly on their genitals.

Alternative massages

There are lots of different ways of giving massage apart from the traditional oil-on-skin methods. For instance, you can bring other tactile sensations into play by deploying your hair, feathers, or soft silky fabrics or scarves on your partner's body. Some of these can be surprisingly effective at relieving stress –

the lightest of touches with a feather brushed over the skin, for example, can swiftly counteract the stresses of everyday life and lead to deepening levels of pleasurable surrender.

You can also treat your partner to a breath massage, or mouth-and tongue massage. Evidently, if you're going to try a feather/mouth/breath massage then you need to start with this before you lead on to other kinds of massage which will require oils.

Be creative: start with a mouth massage and just keep going into a full body massage, or begin with a feather massage combined with a breath massage, then flow into a genital massage. It's up to you – the most important thing is to be giving loving energy to each other.

Massage basics

- Switch off mobiles, banish distractions and lock the door (as I recommend for all sex dates, not just massage).

- The most practical container for oil is a small plastic bottle, which might not look pretty but it's less easily knocked over than a bowl. Warm up the oil bottle beforehand in a basin of hot water.

- Keep a large towel handy to cover the parts of the body not being immediately massaged.

- Add oil to your own hands, not directly onto the body.

- Try to keep your hands in contact with your partner's body, moving as smoothly as you can from one area to the next without lifting them up. If you need to reach for more oil, keep one hand or the side of your arm resting on your partner's body.

- Treat the body symmetrically, spending equal time on each arm, leg, shoulder etc. Don't wander aimlessly around or skip abruptly from one area to the next.

- Spend at least 15-20 minutes on the back – this will help the rest of the body to relax.

- The circulation stroke is easy to learn: moving your hands up the limbs or the chest or back, mould the whole hand to the shape of your partner's body as you go upwards and then draw back down again with a light touch of the fingertips.

- Kneading is another important stroke: make circular movements with your hand, picking up a fold of flesh with your thumb and squeezing gently before letting it go at the end of the circle. Now alternate with your other hand at the same place, so each hand is complementing the other in a smooth, rhythmic motion which will feel continuous to your partner. On fleshy areas, use the whole hand to knead and squeeze.

- Avoid talking unless to quietly ask for feedback along the lines of 'does that feel good?' or 'harder or softer?'

- Most people love to be touched, so don't worry if you haven't mastered any techniques – just create a warm, unhurried space for contact.

- Try mixing and matching different massage techniques. For instance, try feather stroking and kissing at the same time, or blowing and fingertips, or licking and feathering combined. That way you can cover more skin with different types of touch, and turn the sensual dial up to the maximum.

- It's good to rest between massages, so that the first giver has time to relax and the first receiver has time to absorb the benefits of the massage before becoming active as the giver. Ideally keep contact. Either lie side-by-side or lie head-to-toe with your hands cupping each other's genitals.

The feather massage

Choose long, delicate feathers such as peacock or ostrich feathers; the latter are particularly effective since each feather consists of a plume of millions of separate wispy filaments (ostrich feather dusters cost about £15 on-line).

Start by getting your partner to lie down, and begin by stroking the feather(s) gently around the head, shoulders and throat, moving all the way down the body and back up again. The receiver can vocalize their appreciation of the sensations on their body, as well as moving slowly and turning sensuously towards the feather, welcoming the touch on parts of the body where you want more.

"I started our sex date feeling overwhelmed and stressed (too many things to do and think about for work). This date absolutely fit my inner tempo. After our greeting of hearts with 'namaste', my boyfriend asked me to lie down and then started by 'dusting off' my stress off with a feather duster – it literally felt as though my stress was falling away as he worked up and down my body so softly and lightly. The next treat in store for me was a full body massage, and again I felt so grateful to find my stress dissolving as he offered me so much of his loving attention".

Sarah, 61, Manchester.

Mouth and tongue massage

Use your mouth and tongue to explore as much of your partner's body as you can – start with small kisses, applying a little suction as you move over the body. Move on to long, loving licks and then vary the

pace every now and again with 'snake bite' kisses –
flicking the end of your tongue rapidly back and forth
on your partner's skin. Suck on digits – toes and
fingers – but go easy around the toes, they're often
hugely charged with energy and you need to be very
gentle.

You can't expect to lick or kiss every single part of
your lover's body – unless you're very dedicated – but
you should try and cover most areas, not simply going
for the obvious erogenous zones. You can space out
your kisses or licks on larger areas of flesh, perhaps
spending more time on unexpected places which may
turn out to be surprisingly sensitive – the backs of the
knees, behind the ears, around the hairline, or the
crook of the elbow, for instance. Nipples, foreheads,
throats are also very sensitive – as of course are your
partner's genitals.

- Don't use oil beforehand. Take a shower or
  bath as usual but don't dry off completely so
  the skin is damp. As usual, make sure the
  room is very warm so that the recipient
  doesn't get cold.

- If you take your time you will feel tiny
  electrical currents in your tongue as you reach
  places on your partner's body where the
  energy is being generated: you can also try
  visualizing energy as sparks jumping out from
  your tongue on to your lover's body.

- You can also use your teeth – but *very, very*
  gently! Think of an animal mother picking up

its offspring in her mouth – you want to just squeeze with the lightest of touches on fleshy areas.

The breath massage

In this massage you use your breath to erotically stimulate your lover's energy body, exhaling by blowing softly with your mouth about an inch or so above your partner's skin. Begin at the base of the spine, blowing from their buttocks all the way up to the head, then back down again and along their outstretched legs. Repeat three times and then get them to turn over, and start blowing from the heart down to the navel and from the navel down to the genitals.

"Breathe in the fire energy around their genitals, inhaling your lover's sexual heat. Let it fill your being, nourishing you, then blow this hot energy back over their body so your exhalation caresses the belly, top of the breasts, throat, lips and finally the forehead. Now that you have enlivened the principal energy centres that link sex, heart and the psyche, explore by blowing on different parts of your lover's body. Play with your breath over their fingertips, earlobes, nape of the neck and inside of the knees".

Cassandra Lorius *Tantric Secrets.*

The genital massage

After prolonged breathing, kneading, feathering, and anything else you've been giving to your partner you can move into a full-body massage or a genital massage. Equally, if the stroking of your well-oiled hands has led your partner to become aroused then you may also want to keep pleasuring them all the way to climax. You can do this in your usual way or slow it down a little, and continue the stroking until it becomes a genital massage – if your partner is ready for it.

Male to female genital massage

Watch her body language – if her thighs are opening and hips lifting slightly, she's probably receptive to you switching the focus to her genitals. Otherwise, always ask. Remember also to switch to a water-based lubricant.

- Begin by kneeling or standing on her left side (if you're right-handed) facing her feet. Place the palm of one hand over her mound with your fingers reaching around to her perineum. Slide your whole hand up and over her vulva, replacing it with your other hand as you stroke up to her navel. Use a really light touch to maximise her pleasure.

- Place the whole hand over the public area and gently vibrate and then hold. Repeat several times.

- Next, explore the vaginal lips by spreading them open and caressing the insides with your lubricated fingers, then take the labia and press them gently together, squeezing and moving backwards and forward between the perineum and the clitoral hood. Softly tease and caress the clitoris as your hands move over her mound.

- Now move on to more direct stimulation of the clitoris, rolling it between your thumb and index finger and kneading very, very gently up and down either side of her clit. Try different variations – using circular motions with one finger, whilst pressing or squeezing with your thumb. Use two, three, or four fingers with different digits massaging and caressing different areas. This is bound to produce an ecstatic result!

- A variation is to turn around, kneeling between her legs, and still maintaining touch, place your hand palm-forward on her pubic mound, slowly sliding your thumb into her vagina. Grip firmly with your thumb pressing on the top of her vaginal wall and then move your whole arm and hand in a steady rhythm, but not too quickly (aim for massage rather than masturbation speed). After twenty seconds or so release the pressure and move your hand around slightly to the right. Repeat the movements and keep going until you have worked your way around to near the perineum. Unless you are double-jointed you'll find it hard to continue in the same pattern, so either switch to using several fingers (and the same technique) or the thumb on your other hand. As a variation on the above, use both thumbs, going in opposite directions.

- Finally, your partner may be begging you to bring her to orgasm with your usual hand technique – and if you don't have one, now is a good time to learn exactly what that might be. Verbal encouragement and/or showing him how you like are the best way to go.

If this was a tantric genital massage it would involve bringing her to the peak of excitement (but not coming) many times, with rests in between for her to absorb the energy back into her body.

Female to male genital massage

This may sound like a bit of a done deal – it's all visible, so how hard can it be to massage a man's genitals? Women massaging men often end up giving them a hand-job to orgasm, and men virtually never complain. But the same message applies for women handling men as it does for men massaging women – slow down, be tender, take your time, tease it out. Taking on board a few of the strokes below will help create more peaks – and more pleasure.

- With your partner lying on his back and you kneeling between his legs facing him, slide both your oiled and warmed hands from his thighs to his chest and back again. Do this for half-a-dozen strokes. Use long, slow strokes.

- Move towards the area around the genitals, the thighs, hips and stomach, without touching them. Move around to his side and place your hand on his scrotum with the heel of your palm on the underside of his penis and the fingers of the same hand cradling the balls. With the other hand dribble some warm oil over your fingers so that it filters down to his genitals.

- Stroke your hands up and over his balls and penis from the perineum, alternating one hand with the other and making sure that you always keep your hands in contact with your partner's body. This is the reverse of the stroke described for women (above), so it's easy for you both to master this one in the same session.

- A variation on this is to make a V-shape with your thumb and forefinger, massaging upwards over his balls and penis very gently with the palm of your hand. The thumb and forefinger move around the outside of his genitals as the palm slides over the top. Form the thumb and forefinger into a semi-circle holding the top of his scrotum, with your palm resting on his balls. Place the other hand next to it, resting on the base of his penis. Move your hands in opposite directions, gently pulling his balls downwards in one direction whilst stroking his penis upwards in the other direction. You can do these strokes simultaneously or alternate them one after the other, trying to maintain a smooth, flowing motion.

- Place one of your hands on the topside of his penis, between the shaft and his belly. Stroke upwards from the base of the shaft, lifting the penis as you go so that by the time you reach the top it is pointing out at an angle from his body. Alternating your hands, keep stroking upwards from the base, and allowing his cock to fall back slightly to let the next hand catch it on the way up. Following on from this stroke, repeat the same motions except with your hands fully encircling his penis. Slide gently upwards, completing the movement with a slight twist as your hand nears the top. Alternate hands so that it seems like one fluid motion. You could also try the same stroke in reverse.

- Hold the base of the penis. Rest the fingertips of your other hand on the head with the fingers pointing downward. Rotate your fingers, moving them smoothly up and down the shaft. Move them clockwise a few times, then anticlockwise. Alternatively, you can repeat this technique this using the palm of your hand instead of your fingertips.

- Another variation is to grasp the shaft firmly, but not tightly, with both hands and twist your hands gently in opposite directions.

The Nuru massage

A nuru massage is a full body-to-body sensual massage using a special slippery gel. This is a really sensational erotic massage – if you've never tried it before, you'll be left wondering how on earth you got so far in life without having done so! It does require some costs for the special gel and a small investment in some kind of waterproof airbed or polyurethane sheets – but it's worth it. As a juicy sex treat for your partner it's hard to beat.

As essential ingredient is the nuru gel itself. This is a colourless, tasteless and odourless gel made from seaweed, sometimes with other added ingredients such as chamomile. It's a natural gel, and safe to use as a sex lubricant.

The idea is to give your partner a body-to-body massage using this gel - the word nuru is Japanese for slippery or smooth, so you get some idea of the erotic potential.

Nuru massage basics

First, you need to obtain a soft plastic air mattress or a polyurethane (PU) sheet and set them up in the bedroom or other location – in Japan steam rooms are considered ideal. The room needs to be kept very warm, so pre-heat it if necessary. Spread some old towels or other covering around the bed or airbed to stop you worrying about gel splashing everywhere. You can also place one across the head of the airbed.

Next, get everything else you want ready – you're going to take a bath and come out wet, so for obvious reasons you need to set up music, light candles and so forth beforehand.

Now for a long, sexy soak with your partner in the bathtub, Jacuzzi, or under the shower. Warm up the bottle of nuru gel – either in the bath with you or in a separate basin. When you're ready to come out, make sure you stay wet! Make your way to the airbed, pour some of the contents of the nuru gel bottle into a bowl, and add a small quantity of hot water.

The massage

As the masseuse, you're now ready to start slathering the warmed-up gel all over your partner and yourself. When you've both fully covered, you can let your imagination take over with as much body-to-body contact as you can handle. You will want to switch roles and take it in turns to be on top, deliciously slipping and sliding all over and around your partner's body. Trust me, you won't want to stop!

- Gel websites will tell you to use an entire 16oz bottle per massage, but this isn't necessary. Half a bottle per massage is plenty.

- Similarly, buying a special 'wooden nuru massage bowl' is nice but not necessary: any large bowl will do.

- Since the gel is water-soluble it will lose its slippery consistency if you add too much water, so just add a little to start with.

- If you're using a fan heater to warm up the room, don't leave it operating near to you when doing the massage because it will dry out the gel. For safety reasons, turn it off before you emerge dripping from the bath.

- Seaweed wraps are known for their cleansing and detoxifying properties, so there's no need to wash the gel off afterwards. Simple put on a robe and let your skin get the benefit of all the minerals in the seaweed as it dries off.

- Your airbed or PU sheets can similarly be left to dry out, and wiped off with a damp cloth once the water has evaporated.

Nuru supplies

A good place to start is www.numagel.co.uk, which sells 250ml bottles of nuru gel for around £10. They also have some excellent airbeds and good value PU sheets. You can also get a fantastic range of different coloured polyurethane (PU) sheets from www.betweenthesheets.com.

"I had a pretty good idea that my wife would love this massage: she loves hot baths, she loves oils and lotions (like most women I guess…) so I thought it would probably be a success. I put a foam mattress on the bedroom floor and covered it with a double black upvc sheet. Then I warmed the bottle of gel in our very hot, foamy bath. After a sexy, flirtatious bath time together we got out and she lay down on the black sheet whilst I slathered the nuru gel all over her. Hey presto – instant result – she loved it! The moans of satisfaction were loud and repeated.

For the next 30 minutes or so we slithered around like a couple of sex-crazed fish, swapping top and bottom a few times and taking it in turns to dip into the bowl of warm gel and slap it around. It was (literally) sensational sex. Penis, buttocks, boobs, thighs, pussy, feet, hands – everything and anything was slipping and sliding in and around every other body part without any inhibitions.

Because of the gel, our actions were frictionless – like sex underwater, or in space maybe – but this also meant that when it came to intercourse (hard to tell, often, where that began or ended) it was difficult to get a grip. I found myself using her shoulders almost like a set of parallel bars, being the only thing I could pull myself up by. It led to an unparalleled orgasm, though, at least 10 out of 10 I would say. I think hers was just as good!"

Michael, 55, Hastings.

Chapter Eight: The Performance Zone – showtime!

There are many different ways of expressing sensuality and intimacy through performance – for instance dancing, stripping, lap-dancing or belly dancing for you and your partner's pleasure, whether together or separately, passively or actively, taking it in turns or simply putting on a show for their juicy pleasure.

As well as getting you out of the usual horizontal sex routine, some form of dance or striptease brings more body movement and fluidity into your interactions, giving you different ways to express your sexuality, to show appreciation for your partner, or to be creative in connecting with them. It releases sexual energies, freeing up your inner Eros.

It also gives you both the opportunity to explore exhibitionism in a safe environment, to take pride in your body, to show off sexy underwear, and to push your own limits – if you want. Fantasies and role-playing can also be part of a sexy dance or strip session.

So there's no excuse – pencil a sexy performance date into your calendar as soon as possible!

Sensual dancing

Dancing often forms part of courtship rituals. But unless you carry on clubbing or join a local tango class, many couples let this enjoyable form of erotic activity slip by.

Why not enjoy this powerful and intimate way of connecting through dance and movement – a sensual dance session at home allows you to enjoy each other in a way which you may have forgotten. And if you enjoy dancing together in public, then a private, at-home session gives you scope to let your hair down and let the dance take you to its natural conclusion (in a way which you might get arrested for if you did it in public!).

- Prepare the room with romantic lighting, candles or whatever is to your taste. Low lighting is helpful if you're feeling self-conscious.

- Dress appropriately – loose and flowing, or tight and sexy, depending on your mood.

- Let yourself go into the music, allowing your instincts to take over.

- Take it in turns to dance for your lover's pleasure, whilst they watch. Be playful or seductive, and surrender to the music.

Tantric dancing

In Tantric traditions, your sexual energy (or *kundalini*) is usually pictured as a coiled snake which lies sleeping at the base of the spine. The idea of the Snake Dance is to free up this energy and allow the full expression

143

of your sexuality as it moves upwards through your entire body.

- Choose exotic (and preferably instrumental) music with a strong beat.

- Shake out any tensions in your body, and then begin tracing circles with your hips in a long, slow, figure-of-eight movement.

- Envisage the snake at the base of your spine slowly uncoiling and making its way up your spine.

- Reach out to your partner, allowing your snake energies to intertwine and dance a sexy dance together.

Strip joint

Stripping for your partner can be hugely juicy. As well as being a treat for the passive (viewing) partner it's also fun for the stripper: taking off your clothes to please your partner can be very empowering (and arousing) for both of you. So reach down and unleash the sexy beast within! Dare to be exciting, and juicy sex will surely follow.

Most of us are going to have similar issues around body image - not many guys have bodies like the Chippendales and not many women resemble female strippers in the movies either. But then remember *The Full Monty*, a movie about ordinary blokes in all their glorious forms – short, tall, thin, fat, whatever – who end up putting on a strip show. What made them sexy was their attitude, their willingness to 'give it a go' despite all their doubts and insecurities - and their bravery in baring all in public (which you don't have to do!).

"Regardless of whether you're a woman or man stripping for a female partner or audience, if you convey eroticism and confidence, you'll be a hit. In fact, you may have a special advantage – lots of women have never been the recipients of this kind of focussed erotic attention. You may find your girlfriend as easy to whip into a voyeuristic frenzy as those gals who go to watch the Chippendales".

Carole Queen *Exhibitionism for the Shy*.

Strip club:

- Set the scene with candles or soft lighting. Pick some atmospheric music and - whether it's a slow sexy chanteuse or a scorching track with a techno beat – make sure it will last longer than one track.

- Choose clothes without too many tricky fastenings. For her a blouse, skirt, bra, panties, stockings, and high heels are obvious man pleasers.

- For him a suit and tie are good (it gives you more to take off), perhaps with a jockstrap or thong underneath.

- Begin by settling your partner down, perhaps giving your lover some passionate kisses before you start to tease with your striptease.

- Practice first! It will make it much easier, and you will be much more confident, if you do a full dress rehearsal before the event. Take some time when your partner isn't around, put on the clothes or outfit you're going to be using, and do a striptease to your chosen music in front of a mirror.

- Invest in some new lingerie or underwear especially for the strip. For men, a new G-string or thong will make it go with a zing when you get down to that layer. For her, the possibilities are endless: you can push the boundaries with accessories such as nipple tassles, nipple chains, feather clips or other adornments for your breasts (passion8.com has a good selection) or bejewelled G-strings to adorn your pussy when it gets down to that layer.

- Be prepared for just having a laugh. It might all go pear-shaped: whatever happens, keep a playful attitude.

The strip:

FOR HER: Begin dancing, touching yourself, stroking your own breasts and running your hands down your thighs. Pretend it's him who's touching you. Slowly unbutton your blouse, revealing and caressing your breasts. Go to your lover and let them touch your breasts, but pull away quickly and return to your dance. Turn away and remove the blouse, then turn round and throw it to him. Continue to caress yourself. Unzip your skirt and let it fall slowly and seductively to the ground. You might come very close to your partner, turning round so that he watch it slide down over your buttocks. Take off your shoes as suggestively as you can then unroll your stockings, again, throwing them to your lover.

Continue to touch yourself all over as you dance and start to rub your crotch to him know that you're hot. Play with your breasts and slowly remove one bra strap and then the other, turning around to undo the clip. Keeping the bra in place with your hands turn back towards him and then remove the bra altogether. Tease your partner by getting close to him so that he can almost touch your breasts and then pull away. Play with your nipples.

Put your hand into your panties and start to play. Begin to remove your panties, thrusting your bottom in his direction as you do so. You can pull down your panties at the sides to tease before removing them. Take off your garter belt, if you're wearing one, and let it fall. You might writhe on the floor, caressing and stroking yourself, on the floor, bed or chair. If you partner hasn't come to you by then, drape yourself around them and start to tease them with your tongue, lips and whole body until you are both in a passionate frenzy.

FOR HIM: Begin by taking the masculine signatures of life (car keys, wallet, etc) and throwing them down in front of your lover. Slowly and seductively wriggle out of your jacket, throwing it to one side. Next undo your tie slowly and use it to tease her with, perhaps flicking it lightly across her body. Begin to unbutton your shirt, removing it slowly and rubbing it over your body before throwing it to your lover. Keep moving and dancing, but as smoothly as you can take off your shoes and socks. Unbuckle your belt, and tease your partner with it. Run your hands over your body and down into your trousers, making it clear to her that you've got an erection. Unzip your flies and very, very slowly and let the trousers fall to the ground as you continue to touch yourself, running your other hand over your body as you do so. Gyrate in front of your lover, parading your G-string or pouch in front of her face but not letting her touch. If your partner hasn't come to you yet, start to kiss and caress her body until you're both aroused.

Use it all the way in terms of teasing, tantalising, and allowing touching or not –whatever is going to drive your partner the most wild.

"Stripping for your lover can be a wonderful way to boost her sexual interest and provide her with fantasy material for some time to come. You needn't have a perfect, glowing body to entertain her – just dim the lights and strut your stuff. Remember, she probably has a good imagination anyway, so be bold and confident and strip with style".

Glenn Watson *Creative Loveplay*.

Fantasy strip

You could also build in fantasy scenarios if you're going in that direction: Now is the time to spring a surprise on your lover and unleash a fantasy in real life (it could be yours or it could be theirs). Costumes to help you with this are readily available and inexpensive (remember the sex budget?). Stripping schoolgirl, naughty nurse, fantasy fireman, it's all there to play for.

Don't forget that domination and submission roles can also have a part to play in stripping (think girl slave/slave master, or male slave/princess) so use this to the full as you dig down into that reservoir of fantasy and sexuality that we all have inside us.

School for strippers

There are plenty of opportunities if you want to take lessons in stripping, burlesque, belly-dancing or similar performance arts. One of the best know is the London Academy Of Burlesque londonacademyofburlesque.com whose founder Jo King ('Goodtime Mama Jo') says that "it's an exciting visual art form which enables you to express a variety of sexual fantasies and stimulate the essence of your sensuality".

Like stripping, pole dancing is another fantastic way to boost your sexual confidence and turn your partner on at the same time. You can indulge your exhibitionist fantasies and prepare to become your lover's very own 'private dancer'. Classes are available through Polestars polestars.net and My Pole Dance School (mypole.co.uk). Pole systems and other accessories are also available from on-line retailers such as lovehoney.co.uk

Belly dancing is a great celebration of womanhood, even thought it's not usually as erotica-oriented as stripping. There are a huge number of different styles of belly dancing: for more info and classes check out bellydancer.org.uk.

Chapter Nine: Becoming Kinky

We've come a long way since the dictionary definition of kinky was closer to sexual perversion rather than simply enjoying a sexual diversion or two and exploring the erotic charge of our deeper desires. This normalisation has been going on for quite some time, with shops, websites, and clubs devoted to kinky fetishes and fantasies springing up everywhere. Retail outlets such as London's Coco de Mer have also taken aspects of kinky sex upmarket with their promotion of wonderful designer toys or props catering for all kinds of erotic play. It has also propelled itself into the general population with the huge global success of the *Fifty Shades of Grey* trilogy.

Definitions

Under the general umbrella of 'BDSM' lie: bondage and discipline (B&D), dominance and submission (D&S) and sado-masochism (S&M). They are all linked because the activities that take place in each also take place, to a greater or lesser extent, in the others. BDSM is very often made up of 'scenarios' where you must decide not only who is to be dominant but if there are further roles to play, what are these and how will they affect sex play, so Fantasy is also important.

Bondage

The 'soft' end of the kinky spectrum, fun to explore in a gentle way but obviously there are people who go to extraordinary lengths to create different (and often bizarre) types of bondage situation. Each to their own

– and you don't have to get into the extremes of bondage fetishism to enjoy a little light sex play with restraints and cuffs.

Bondage is arousing because, paradoxically, restraints can act as a release for your inhibitions and being controlled - or in control – can be wildly exciting. Men enjoy being tied down because it allows them the freedom to be more passive than they usually are during sex. Women also enjoy the sense of helplessness when they're tied but, equally, can revel in the sexual freedom of being totally in control when it's their partner who's tied down.

For either partner it's a surrender to domination, a state of vulnerability which allows you to concentrate on and give in to the potentially very intense sensations of being pleasured.

Bondage requires (and creates) trust between partners. All bondage and discipline activities should be strictly consensual. It's very important that you agree on a code word before you begin that will indicate that your partner is not enjoying what you are doing to them. Remember, your partner is unable to move so must be able to communicate to you. Often in the heat of passion the word 'stop' can be interpreted as 'please keep doing that'. So it's best to choose another word, such as 'Red'. Never leave your partner alone and tied. If you have to leave the room for a minute, tell them that you will be back. Always make your partner feel safe.

If you've never tried this before, begin with a small suggestive action, such as holding your partner's wrists, or stretching them out above their head and holding them during lovemaking. If you decide to move from here, use silk scarves, belts or ties while you experiment and find what you like.

By now you and your partner should be able to talk about what you like and you can both shop for more expensive restraining goods. Basic handcuffs (metal or plastic) can be cheap, but really it's better to invest in something of good quality. Leather cuffs have a sensual attraction but generally cuffs can come in all types materials including "fluffy fur" cuffs. Even the way in which the cuffs are fastened can be important—velcro-fastened cuffs are easy to attach and remove whereas buckle cuffs add to the thrill of restraint which is difficult to escape from.

If you have two sets then use one set to hook either wrists or ankles (arms or legs splayed) to the bed head, four sets will allow you to attach your partner to all four corners of the bed.

Another option is bondage tape, which is a reusable pvc tape that only sticks to itself and won't cling to your skin, clothes or even hair. It can also be easily and painlessly removed. Bind your partner to you or to the bed, furniture or themselves, but remember to use it safely and wisely.

The most popular position for tying up your lover is spread-eagled on a bed, tied at wrists and ankles (facing up or facing down, depending upon how you are going to develop your sex play). Facing up allows the 'love-giver' access to chest, breast, genitals, head and neck area of their lover. Facing down allows for massage, anal penetration, and spanking. Experiment and see what you both like. If your bed has a footboard, you might want to tie up the passive partner lying sideways across the bed to give better access. Tying wrists or arms behind backs or behind the neck can let the recipient experience the sensuality of restraint without being completely immobile, allowing you and your partner to change positions or move from room to room. Another variation is to tie wrists to ankles (usually behind the back) giving the receiver further sensation as they move and wriggle, knowing that they are tied to themselves. There is plenty of opportunity to use props in order to enjoy the experience of different positions, such as, tying your lover to the kitchen chair or binding their hands so that they are leaning over a desk or table.

If you are the dominant lover, that is, you are not the one who is tied, you will find it easy to think of ways to tease your partner after you realise that they are at your mercy. Remember to tell them so because talking can be part of the arousal. Stimulate your partner enough to keep them excited all the time, bring them up to a high state of arousal then lower it again to prolong the pleasure.

"Imagination is the key to good sex. I defy anyone not to enjoy at least bondage (with no discipline). It is a wonderful feeling to be strapped down and made love to because you don't have to think about anything—just relax and enjoy the sensations'.

Jo-Anne Baker (Ed) *Sex Tips from Women Who Ride The Sexual Frontier.*

- Tease your partner by caressing, massaging, stroking, licking or even masturbating yourself.

- Use feathers, sexy fabrics, vibrators, bedroom foods, ice cubes or sensual oils.

- Remember to keep in contact with your partner as much as possible even if it is just resting a hand on their body. If you partner is tied and blindfolded then occasionally move away for a few seconds (but stay in the room) because the thrill of not knowing which part of their sensitised body is going to be touched next will excite your partner.

- Use your body oil and rub yourself—all of you, or just parts of you—against your partner, for example using your fingers and toes or your genitals.

- You might want to try a striptease, running items of clothing—stockings, knickers or scarves—over your partner's body and genitals as you remove them.

Blindfolds are a natural part of bondage games because it makes the passive partner more helpless and creates great suspense. Either make your next move a surprise or sexily whisper exactly what you're going to do into their ear. For example, you might want to introduce a new vibrator this way buzzing it next to their ear to begin with before moving on to their body. The thrill of knowing that something very pleasurable is going to happen, but not knowing what it is or where it will happen, can be a great turn-on.

Bondage is very much part of the next two sections on fantasy, bondage and discipline, and dominance and submission. Don't be afraid to experiment and mix up all these different techniques including them in more general creative sex play.

"Sex is supposed to pack a punch. It's supposed to take you off guard, make you hold your breath for what might come next, gasp with discovery, quicken your pulse and consume you, mind, body and soul. Sexual desire should make you say and do things that you would never normally do, and the severity and physical sensations should paralyse you. Sex should set you on fire, so that an unrecognizable shade of yourself comes alive in the smolder".

Debra & Don Macleod *Fifty Ways to Play*

Bondage and discipline

Bondage and discipline involves restraint and some form of discipline, either verbal or using toys such as whips or paddles. Examples of discipline can include light spanking or using whips or paddles, and verbal discipline, such as 'you've been a bad boy, you won't be getting that treat that I promised you'. One partner is submissive and one partner is dominant (see D&S below). You don't have to go down the route of extremes to enjoy a little mischief in your sex games and have tough and tender fun at the same time.

Although plenty of couples enjoy the balance of pleasure and pain that comes with BDSM, many others will simply be content with a little erotic spanking, which increases blood flow to the genital regions and highlights the sexual sensations.

If you never tried bondage and discipline before, start by simply tying up your partner and pleasuring them. From here you can move on to use a little discipline as part of sex play, for example, introduce light slapping of the buttocks. The line between pleasure and pain is a fine one so be gentle and listen to your partner's reactions until you find out what they like. Remember that you can mix B&D in with all and any kind of sex play including massage, touching and stroking, penetration, etc. Do keep reassuring your partner that they can use the 'stop' codeword whenever they want to.

You can basically spank with just your hand, or introduce other objects which will add to the sense of novelty. You could start with a lightweight rubber whip (known as a 'pussy' or 'cock' whips), which can be trailed across your partner's body and genitals and occasionally used for a gentle beating. You can graduate to leather whips and paddles or a spanking rod if you feel comfortable with this.

Adopting a stern, forbidding voice will add to the authority figure role, and you can admonish your lover this way: "You've been a very, very bad girl", uttered in a threatening whisper. Your partner might join in with melodramatic pleas for mercy and promises not to repeat the offence—these are all part of the game. You might want to adopt aliases for your favourite roles, so that each of you can indicate to your partner when you want to play that game simply by using that particular name.

Browse online sex shops for inspiration about what type of toys you might like to buy. If you're thinking about punishment scenarios, ensure that they are make-believe. You shouldn't be expressing real anger.

"The pleasure-loving side of us...will take different forms in different people, for none of us develops alike in our eroticism any more than in our physical bodies. For some, the erotic self emerges as a stud or bombshell; in others it is as playful as a child. In some it will be imperious and dominant; in others it will be eager to please. For many of us, a number of erotic archetypes lie under the surface of our personalities, waiting to be asked out to play".

Carol Queen *Exhibitionism for the Shy.*

Dominance and submission

Dominance and submission means that one partner (submissive) follows the will of the other partner (dominant) and can include simple bondage (tying up) or an extreme form of bullying (making your partner walk around on all fours wearing a dog collar and licking your boots). The latter is a world of sexual servitude with 'tops' (those in control) and 'bottoms' (those being controlled), and power games. However, you must ensure that both parties in this game enjoy what they are doing.

You can bring mild D&S into the bedroom, ordering your partner to carry out your wishes, such as, to fuck you, suck you, or simply to lick your toes. Begin with small, short tasks during regular sex play. You might find that it's a good way to introduce new skills or new techniques that you want to try. When you graduate to one partner being fully in control, then they can order their partner to pleasured them or they can pleasure their partner.

- One of the simplest and most effective sub/dom games is the reward/punishment scenario of not letting your partner move or respond while you pleasure them. For instance, you give your partner oral sex, causing them to writhe in pleasure. But you order them not to move, which will create the most exquisite tension in your partner, who is longing to respond to your caresses and touch but is forced to sublimate desires.

- This probably works best with oral or manual stimulation of your partner's genitals, but it could also include occasional penetration to sustain arousal.

- You can also tie them down and tease him/her with a vibrator, for instance with the male dominant inserting a vibrator into the vagina of his tied-down partner, who is forced to climax as she writhes in sexual ecstasy. She may well push herself harder and harder onto the vibrator in an effort to come – which he can deny, pulling it away to tantalise her and prolong her agony.

- Female dominants can also force their male submissive to masturbate in front of them, or insist on masturbating in front of him (possibly *very* close up) without him being allowed to touch him – or her.

- She can also use a penis pump or male masturbator on him, to bring him to climax or as close to climax as she wants.

As previously noted, you inevitably mix up these techniques with each other and with the rest of your sex play. Tie down your partner and take them to new heights: strip them of control, take over and submit them to a range of sensations though domination including a gentle spanking. As you starting to feel comfortable with what you do, don't be afraid to take your roles, or the punishment that you give, to a slightly higher level. Watch your partner's reactions and find out if they're levels of arousal are changing. Don't be afraid of making mistakes. Remember however, to retain a code word for when you've had enough.

"BDSM sex play can be a mentally and physically exhausting experience. It is absolutely essential that partners care for each other afterward. Men in the role of dominants must be especially careful to comfort and reassure their female partner. For some couples, aftercare involves cuddling and talking to reaffirm the feelings of love between them. For others, aftercare is more about postcoital giggling as they pack up their handcuffs, penis rings and butt plugs. A shared laugh is often more bonding than an embrace"

Debra & Don Macleod *Fifty Ways to Play*

AFTERWORD

I hope you enjoyed reading this book – and putting some of the ideas into practice – as much as my partner and I did in writing it. We also shared it with friends who were kind enough to add their comments to our text.

If you've got this far you'll know by now that it's not really about tricks or techniques but about communication, intimacy, and loving honesty. Small but loving day-to-day actions – kissing your partner when they're least expecting it, hugging them at any time, caressing them without expectations beyond giving pleasure – are vastly more important than positions or expensive lingerie. Being helpful and supportive – taking on household chores, sharing problems, listening deeply – are also key in any loving relationship. This is an attitude, along with an open mind and an willingness to explore boundaries, which will ensure you'll continue to enjoy juicy sex well into the prime of your lives and beyond.

Further reading

A Beginner's Guide to Tantric Sexuality by Richard Craze (Hodder & Stoughton 1999).

A Piece of Cake: Recipes for Female Sexual Pleasure by Melinda Gallagher and Emily Scarlet Kramer (Atria Books 2005).

Creative Loveplay by Dr Glenn Wilson (Carrol & Graff 1996),.

Exhibitionism for the Shy: Show Off, Dress Up and Talk Hot by Carol Queen (Down There Press 1995).

Fifty Shades of Bliss: The Ultimate Guide to Spicing up Your Sex Life by Lexie Sutton (Summersdale 2012).

Fifty Ways to Play: A Beginner's Guide to UnleashingYour Erotic Desires by Debra Macleod and Don Macleod (Harper 2012).

Hot Sex by Tracey Cox (Corgie Books 1998).

How to Tell a Naked Man What to Do by Candida Royale (Piatkus 2004).

Lesbian Sex Secrets for Men by Jamie Goddard and Kurt Brungardt (Penguin 2000).

Make Love Like a Prairie Vole: Six Steps to Passionate, Plentiful and Monogamous Sex by Andrew G Marshall (Bvloomsbury 2012).

Sensational Sex: the Revolutionary Guide to Sexual Pleasure and Fulfilment by Dr Pam Spurr (Robson Books 2006).

Sex Talk: How to Tell Your Lover Exactly What You Want, Exactly When You Want It by Carole Altman (Sourcebooks 2004).

Sex Tips from Women who Ride the Sexual Frontier by Jo-Anne Baker (Fusion Press 2000).

Sexual Ecstasy: The Art of Orgasm by Margot Anand (Penguin Putnam 2000).

Sexual Intelligence by Dr Sheree Conrad & Dr Michael Milburn (Crown Publishers 2001).

Tantra: The Art of Mind-Blowing Sex by Val Sampson (Vermilion 2002).

Tantric Secrets: 7 Steps to the Best Sex of your Life by Cassandra Lorius. (Thorsons 2003).

The Art of Sensual Massage by Gordon Inkeles and Murray Todris (George Allen & Unwin 1973).

The Barefoot Doctor's Handbook for Modern Lovers by Stephen Russell (Piatkus 2000).

The Clitoral Truth by Rebecca Chalker (Seven Stories Press 2000).

The Enlightened Sex Manual by David Deida (Sounds True 2004).

The Joy of Sex by Alex Comfort (Quartet Books 1996).

The Sexual Teachings of the Jade Dragon by His Lai (Destiny Books 2002).

Ultimate Undies Eds Rachel Kramer Bussek and Christopher Pierce (Alyson Books 2006).

5 Minutes to Orgasm Every Time You Make Love by D.Claire Hutchins (JPS Publishing 2000).

226 Ways to Unleash the Sex Goddess in Every Woman by Olivia St Claire (Bantam 1996).